Access your online resources

Music, Sound and Vibration in Special Education is accompanied by a number of printable online materials, designed to ensure this resource best supports your professional needs.

Activate your online resources:

* Go to www.routledge.com/cw/speechmark and click on the cover of this book
* Click the 'Sign in or Request Access' button and follow the instructions in order to access the resources

Music, Sound and Vibration in Special Education

This book provides practical guidance on how to successfully incorporate music, sound and vibration into your special school, exploring the rich benefits that musical opportunities offer for children with physical, mental health and learning disabilities.

Music has been shown to improve mood, lift depression, improve blood flow and even ease pain, whilst musical interventions can encourage communication and enable relaxation. This book explores the physical, cognitive and mental health benefits of music use in special schools, introducing therapies and innovations that can be adapted for use in your own specialist setting.

Key features include:

* Chapters exploring a range of music therapies and technologies that allow all students to access the benefits of music, sound and vibration, from one-to-one therapeutic music sessions to vibro-acoustic therapy and sing and sign
* Case studies and anecdotes showcasing the innovative ways that special schools are using music, and providing concrete examples of how to deliver, record and access music provision
* Photocopiable policies, risk assessments and links to useful resources

Written by an author with a wealth of experience in special education, this book is essential reading for all those working in specialist settings or with children with SEND.

Ange Anderson, M.Ed. is a SEND consultant and advisor for schools, specialising in therapeutic and technological interventions for additional learning needs. She supports schools on site as well as remotely through Teams and Zoom meetings. She is the special needs advisor for an international VR company. She is the former headteacher of a leading specialist school and author of special educational books and children's books. She has authored several educational articles and papers on therapeutic intervention, is involved in international research work and has presented internationally on topics related to special education.

Music, Sound and Vibration in Special Education

How to Enrich Your Specialist Setting

Ange Anderson

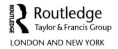

Routledge
Taylor & Francis Group

LONDON AND NEW YORK

First published 2021
by Routledge
2 Park Square, Milton Park, Abingdon, Oxon OX14 4RN

and by Routledge
605 Third Avenue, New York, NY 10158

Routledge is an imprint of the Taylor & Francis Group, an informa business

© 2021 Ange Anderson

British Library Cataloguing-in-Publication Data
A catalogue record for this book is available from the British Library

Library of Congress Cataloging-in-Publication Data
Names: Anderson, Ange, author.
Title: Music, sound and vibration in special education : how to enrich your
    specialist setting with music / Ange Anderson.
Description: [1.] | New York : Routledge, 2021. | Includes bibliographical
    references and index.
Identifiers: LCCN 2020056449 (print) | LCCN 2020056450 (ebook) |
    ISBN 9780367708283 (hardback) | ISBN 9780367708306 (paperback) |
    ISBN 9781003148173 (ebook)
Subjects: LCSH: Special education. | Music therapy. | Sound—Therapeutic use. |
    Vibration—Therapeutic use.
Classification: LCC MT17 .A6 2021 (print) | LCC MT17 (ebook) |
    DDC 371.9/04487—dc23
LC record available at https://lccn.loc.gov/2020056449
LC ebook record available at https://lccn.loc.gov/2020056450

ISBN: 978-0-367-70828-3 (hbk)
ISBN: 978-0-367-70830-6 (pbk)
ISBN: 978-1-003-14817-3 (ebk)

Typeset in Optima
by Apex CoVantage, LLC

Access the companion website: www.routledge.com/cw/speechmark

Dedication

This book is dedicated to special schools everywhere that use music, sound and vibration to educate and enhance the lives of their students.

Contents

Contents

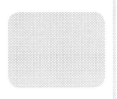

Figures

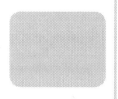

Tables and downloadable resources

Acknowledgements

I would like to thank all the staff of the special schools that appear in this book. I would particularly like to thank Gavin Shakespeare, the current therapist in music at Ysgol Pen Coch for his detailed response to my queries and also Toni Bailey, Assistant Director for Peterborough and Cambridgeshire, responsible for SEND and inclusion who was able to give me a local authority view on the impact on EHC plan provision during the course of the pandemic.

I would like to thank Future Education business manager, Mark Anderson, for his input on how teenagers with complex needs have been analysing the effects of music on their lives.

Special thanks go to Jonathan Bryan for allowing me to include his very moving poem in the introduction and also to Cheryl Galea, the holistic sound practitioner at Ysgol Y Deri for the inclusion of one of her sound therapy sessions in chapter 5.

I would also like to thank the headteachers who gave up their time to discuss or correspond with me on the impact the pandemic had on their school. They are Chris Britten, head of Ysgol Y Deri in Penarth; Noel Fitzgerald, head of Ysgol Pen Coch in Flint; Julian Lewis, assistant head of Ysgol Pen Coch in Flint; Donna Roberts, head of Ysgol Hafod Lon in Penrhydeudraeth; Andreas Huws, head of Ysgol y Bont in Anglesey; Jonathan Morgan, head of Ysgol Gogarth in Llandudno; and Rhona O'Neil, head of Ysgol Tir Morfa in Rhyl.

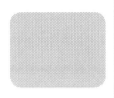

Abbreviations

AAC	Alternative and Augmentative Communication
ADHD	Attention Deficient Hyperactive Disorder
AIT	Auditory Integration Training
AMT	Adaptive Music Technology
AMTRG	Adaptive Music Technology Research Group
APMT	Association of Professional Music Therapists
ARR	Assessment, Recording and Reporting
ARROW	Aural Read Respond Oral Write
ASC	Autistic Spectrum Condition
ASD	Autism Spectrum Disorder
ASL	American Sign Language
BAMT	British Association for Music Therapy
BJSE	British Journal of Special Education
BJMT	British Journal of Music Therapy
BSMT	British Society for Music Therapy
BSL	British Sign Language
CCI	Creative Computing Institute
CMA	Complementary Medical Association
CSAM	Connecting Steps Assessment Module
DfE	Department for Education
D-PAN	Deaf Professional Art Network
EBD	Emotional Behavioural Difficulties
EHC	Educational Health Care plan
ENT	Ear, Nose and Throat
FST	Filtered Sound training
HCPC	Health and Care Professional Council
HIFU	High Intensity Focussed Sound
HLTA	Higher level teaching assistant
Hz	Hertz
IAHP	Institute for Achievement of Human Potential

IDP	Individual Development Plan
IEP	Individual Education Plan
LA	Local Authority
MIAV	Music is a vibration
MiSP	Mindfulness in Schools Project
NIH	National Institute of Health
OKMT	Otakar Kraus Music Trust
OPEF	Oscillating Pulsed Electric Field
PMLD	Profound and Multiple Learning Difficulties
POPAT	Programme of Phoneme Awareness Training
PPE	Personal Protection Equipment
PROMISE	Provision of Music in Special Education
RfL	Routes for Learning
SEN	Special Educational Needs
SEND	Special Educational Needs and Disability
SLA	Service Level Agreement
SLD	Severe Learning Difficulties
SOI	Sounds of Intent
SSE	Sign Supported English
TA	Teaching Assistant
UAL	University of the Arts London
UN	United Nations
VAT	Vibro-acoustic therapy

Introduction

In 1999 Ofsted, England's school inspectorate, stated that only one-third of special schools provided music lessons. I feel that this was a misunderstanding by Ofsted of how students encounter sound, vibration and music in special schools that provide for students with a primary diagnosis of severe, complex or profound learning difficulties. It is not always about a scheduled lesson. The importance of music in a special school cannot be undervalued.

Special schools are each made up of students diagnosed with complex learning difficulties and disabilities (CLDD), severe learning difficulties (SLD) and with profound and multiple learning difficulties (PMLD). Each student may also have added conditions such as autism, life threatening illnesses and individual needs.

Students with CLDD have conditions that co-exist, creating a complex profile. These students may have a range of issues such a mental health, behavioural, physical, medical, sensory, communication and cognition. They will need support to enable them to access the curriculum.

If a student cannot participate in the regular aspects of daily life, the disabilities are considered severe and the student is considered as having severe learning difficulties (SLD). They may also have difficulties in mobility and coordination, communication, and the acquisition of self-help skills. They will need support in all areas of the curriculum so that they can learn.

The term profound and multiple disabilities (PMLD) refers to the presence of two or more conditions, each representing a different disability category. This will include the more common disabilities affecting cognition and learning which is usually assessed as profound, as well as the low incidence disabilities of vision impairment, auditory impairment, other health impairments and/or physical disability. Assessing PMLD in children is a challenge due to their language, cognition, sensory and motor abilities which can complicate accurate diagnosis. A student diagnosed with PMLD requires a high level of adult support, both for accessing learning and their personal care, but that does not mean that they cannot learn and should not be given the opportunity to learn.

Students with autism and other conditions attend special schools but only if they have, additionally, SLD, CLDD or PMLD.

All children can academically achieve and the only barrier to learning is lack of expectation. The institute for the achievement of human potential (IAHP) founded in 1955 by Glen Dolman has had many successes over the years in teaching students with a diagnosis of PMLD (Dolman 2005). If you are interested in their research and how they have helped innumerable children diagnosed with PMLD and severe learning difficulties (SLD) to read and to achieve their potential, go to https://www.iahp.org.

I include here a poem written by Jonathan Bryan, diagnosed as having PMLD. He attended both a special school and a mainstream school and strongly supports all children being taught to read and write, regardless of their educational label. He used an E-Tran frame (see Section 1 of the Appendix) for eye pointing to spell out words.

PMLD
We are not capable of learning
So do not tell me
There's something going on behind the disability.
Treated as useless handicaps
Minds with nothing in there, tragically
Stuck in a wheelchair,
Disabilities visibly crippling –
Just incontinent and dribbling,
We are not
Academically able.
You should make our minds
Stagnate in special education!
We cannot
Learn to read,
Learn to spell,
Learn to write,
Instead let us
Be constrained by a sensory curriculum.
It is not acceptable to say
We have the capacity to learn.
School should occupy us, entertain us; but never teach us
You are deluded to believe that
Our education can be looked at another way!
NOW READ THE POEM AGAIN BACKWARDS.

(Bryan 2018)

Please visit www.teachustoo.org.uk to find out more about Jonathan and his charity.

To class a child as having PMLD does not tell you whether that child is deaf or blind or both; whether that child has other sensory impairments; whether that child has Niemann Pick C disease or Cockayne syndrome or West syndrome or Dravet syndrome or Sanfilippo syndrome (see Sections 2, 3, 4, 5 or 6 of the Appendix) or a host of other syndromes – all of which I have encountered in my years in special schools. The appendix will tell you more about how music helped those students. For now, I want to tell you about how music helped a particular student in 2018.

The student had a primary diagnosis of PMLD. He also had albinism and autism. He required the regular assistance of the vision support service and had sensory processing difficulties. He would regularly strip all of his clothes off and rarely wore footwear. He was overweight but he was loved and a very happy child.

When karaoke machines and microphones became all the rage a few years ago we purchased a cheap one to trial. In 2018 his very intuitive caring teacher came to see me to ask if the school would purchase a wireless microphone and karaoke set, as he had noticed the student making noises into the plastic version we had. He had never made noises before and James, the teacher, was excited by the possibility. We purchased the set he asked for.

The student took to the microphone like a duck to water. As long as we gave him a microphone and he could hear the echo of his own voice he would sing whatever he could hear being sung. He had not uttered a word before. He began repeating not just snippets of songs but meaningful words too.

The class teacher began using the set for registration and the student said his name in answer to the register for the first time in the five years he had attended our school. He began to communicate that he needed the toilet. He began to use a TEACCH station. He would sing quietly and use the karaoke machine. The microphone and karaoke machine were the key to his communication. On the Sounds of Intent Framework (see Section 7 of the Appendix) he was performing at a level 6. That is not a PMLD level.

We ended up buying several karaoke machines with microphones for different classes and although they certainly assisted with students' communication, none of them had that same profound effect. Music, sound and vibration, in all their variations, have had equally profound effects on some of our other students.

We have to remember that in a special school it is not about raising standards to enable our students to become part of a workforce. It is about having an appropriate curriculum to meet the needs of the students so that they may make progress according to their needs and desires. It is primarily about enabling them to communicate. Most children have a desire to learn, but most children do not have barriers to learning that first need to be overcome. Students in a special school should be constantly assessed as to how they can best learn so that they achieve their potential, but they also have to have their other needs met. We all know that when we are going through a traumatic personal event we cannot concentrate properly. Imagine having a mind that is in constant turmoil. Imagine having a condition where you are in daily physical pain. Now imagine that you are just a child. It is important that we first ensure that our students are in the right frame of mind to learn. We may accomplish this by offering therapeutic interventions. Often when a person reaches adulthood, they question whether what they learnt in school was useful. In any school education should be relevant. The curriculum should be appropriate to meet the needs of the students and evidence needs to be provided to show progression. Assessment is essential.

Sound, music and vibration are relevant in a special school, but they may not be delivered in the way they are delivered in a mainstream school. I recall a member of staff in a special school showing disapproval when I wanted a student who was deaf to join a music session. Anyone can experience the joy of music and feel the vibrational benefits of sound. Dame Evelyn Glennie has been profoundly deaf since the age of 12, having started to lose her hearing from the age of eight. She has her own YouTube channel, where she states that we all feel sound and that we need to open up our bodies like a resonating chamber. Her videos demonstrate how we can all feel sound. She regularly plays barefoot during both live performances and studio recordings to feel the music better. She demonstrates how anyone, regardless of their disability, can develop musical skills and appreciate music.

Music is used constantly in special schools. It has been used for transition throughout the day in every special school that I have worked in, supported or inspected. Many parents working closely with special school staff also use music to indicate periods of transition at home. Music is an important communication tool. Music is used in therapies, training, dance, literacy, numeracy, PHSE, assemblies and in meditation, and in most other subjects because children with special needs relate to music so well. Music, sound and vibration play a big part in the teaching and learning of special schools. If you follow the video links throughout the book you will get an idea of just how much music is used in a special school.

I feel that the school inspectors in 1999 concentrated on a mainstream model of music education and it is good to see that the curriculum models have moved forward 20 years later to take account of what special schools have been providing. It is merely my opinion but a student performing at a PMLD/SLD/CLDD level does not necessarily require a traditional music lesson over other sessions and activities that encompass music, sound or vibration. These can meet the student's individual targets better and members of staff will need to remember to use the Sounds of Intent (SOI) Framework (see Section 7 of the Appendix) or indeed Wales' updated Routes for Learning (RfL) Framework (see Section 8 of the Appendix) or England's Engagement Model (see Section 9 of the Appendix) or Ireland's Quest for Learning Model (see Section 10 of the Appendix) – which is based on Wales' Routes for Learning assessment materials published in 2006. This is so that progress in music, sound and vibration can be shown across all subjects, because music is used in most subjects and therapies and it may be worthwhile showing off to the inspectorate the true amount of musical activity students in a special school encounter and respond to every day.

As you will see through reading this book, some students do require one-to-one music sessions, some students require therapeutic music or music as part of another therapy, and all students require the opportunity to sing and sign. A highlight for many schools is a visiting musician in residence or maybe a band. I well remember us having the whole of a local male voice choir attend our school and perform for us. We also regularly performed with other special schools at the local cathedral where the acoustics were amazing. A special school could not manage without music at its core. It is time special schools were valued for the usually intense amount of musical opportunities on offer. Perhaps special schools were just not advertising what they do enough when Ofsted visited in 1999.

I have no doubt that special schools vary in the ways that they deliver, record and assess their provision of music, vibration and sound. There may be some teachers, parents, carers or indeed inspectors who require guidance on what is available. This book is written for them.

1 | What is therapeutic music in a special school setting?

The therapeutic value of music

Daniel Levitin, author of *This Is Your Brain on Music* (2019), found that music activates more areas of the brain than language. It creates more neural activity and more electrical firing reaches into greater crevices.

Not all sound is music. Yet all music is sound. Music is sound that has order and pattern. We can relate to order and pattern. I know I feel the need for order in my life and pattern exists in every phase of our lives as well as in nature and indeed the universe. Is that why I love music so much? Does it fill a need in me? In Darwin's book *The Descent of Man and Selection in Relation to Sex* – published in 1871 – he hypothesises that the second stage in man's development of language (the first being development of cognitive ability) was the development of a musical protolanguage (Fitch 2009). This suggest that music has always played an important role in the development of man.

Therapeutic music is music that is used to aid the mental and emotional well-being of those listening or partaking in the music experience. Music therapy makes use of music in order to address the various spiritual, physical, cognitive, social and emotional needs of individuals belonging to all age groups.

Think about how different music makes you feel mentally, emotionally and physically. You may use up-tempo music for exercise, different types of music for different styles of dance, and calming, soothing music to relax or meditate to. Music affects us psychologically.

Eight years ago, it was a Saturday and I was on my way to school day. I was head of a special school and wanted to get on with some work in my office without being disturbed, and I felt that a Saturday was ideal. As it was a Saturday there was no clock to watch and I should have taken my time. I turned the car radio on, and the radio station was playing 'The flight of the Bumble Bee' by Rimsky Korsakov. As the music got faster so did my driving. I have the shame of being done for speeding on my way to school on a Saturday!

Mark Anderson, business manager at Future Education in Norwich, a school for teenagers with social, emotional and mental health needs, told me how they are working with students on analysing the statistics for music played whilst driving in relation to car accidents. He is keen for Future Education to create a VR environment for students to experience the effects safely so that it informs them for the future when they may drive a car of their own.

Music can and does influence us. I recall dating a professor of music seven years ago who composed a piece of music for me about the walk we had been on for our third date. It sounds romantic, doesn't it? I had certainly enjoyed the walk, which was a guided walk amongst the hills of Snowdonia and had lasted six hours instead of the three advertised. I have to admit that I could see he was struggling towards the end. The piece of music he thoughtfully composed for me can only be described as a dirge. It told me more about his experience that day than words ever could.

We often take the power of music for granted. Sometimes we change the music we are listening to according to need or mood, and if we really think about how and why we have done that, then it becomes easy to understand how it can be used in a therapeutic manner to aid someone suffering with specific issues.

Music Therapists

A school is incredibly lucky if it has the funds for therapeutic music to be delivered by a qualified Music Therapist. Music Therapists have been able to demonstrate breakthroughs in achieving physical, emotional and cognitive responses from people who had seemed inaccessible to other forms of intervention. They build up relationships with their clients and learn what type of music therapy works best. When I was deputy head in a secondary special school, we had a student who was a large six-foot young man and could destroy a classroom in seconds, but every week he would sit quietly for half an hour on his own with the Music Therapist (quite a small woman) and occasionally join in on the piano. For the rest of the day he remained chilled.

Nordoff & Robins developed music therapy for children with psychological, physical and intellectual disabilities in the 1960s, and the charity now trains many Music Therapists in their approaches in England and other countries. There is a professional association – the Association of Professional Music Therapists (APMT). The British Society for Music Therapy (BSMT) publishes the *British Journal of Music Therapy* (*BJMT*). Both the association and the journal are available to support qualified Music Therapists.

Some progressive local authorities employ Music Therapists as part of their music support to schools. I wish I had worked for one of those authorities, but I didn't. Some schools pay for a self-employed registered Music Therapist to visit their school weekly, fortnightly or even monthly depending on what they can afford. Some independent schools employ a registered Music Therapist.

Ockelford et al. (2002) stated in the findings from the PROMISE research project of 2001 that only 2% of students with PMLD or SLD received music therapy. The PROMISE (Provision of Music in Special Education) national survey in England was again completed in 2015. Of the 57 schools that took part, a third of those schools employed a Music Therapist. This suggests that more schools are now managing to deliver music as a therapy. Funding has always been the issue. Let me assure you that if every special school were offered a Music Therapist and they did not have to worry about the funding they would bite your hand off.

When I was deputy head of the secondary special school in 2000, we paid for the Music Therapist to attend one day a week, as it was all we could afford. I have inspected and supported schools recently where this practice still continues. To work as a registered Music Therapist, you must be registered with the Health and Care Professions Council (HCPC). You can only register if you have completed a master's qualification accredited by the British Association for Music Therapy (BAMT) and recognised by the HCPC.

In my experience, the school either chooses the students most in need of the therapy or the student's statement of educational need specifies that the student requires this therapy. This is now known as an educational and health care plan (EHCP) in England. To find out about the change in statementing in other areas of the UK, go to the website https://www.contact.org.uk. All educational care plans, however they are named, are reviewed every year. The school needs to find the funding for this therapy and that may be why many schools have to prioritise – because, in my opinion, every single student benefits from therapeutic music.

A qualified Music Therapist is also able to train school staff or care home staff to continue with the programme they have devised for individuals, making it more cost friendly. It is an invaluable support, as the member of staff has been trained by someone who is qualified and who can assess progress on a weekly, fortnightly or monthly basis, depending on the budget available. If you go to www.musicastherapy.org, you can find out about some of the amazing work Music Therapists do to make music's unique benefits available to as many vulnerable and marginalised people as possible.

When I became head of a new school in 2009, I was genuinely concerned that the school was expected to pay into a music service level agreement (SLA) with the local authority, yet that did not include access to a Music Therapist. The SLA supported the music service in delivery of music across the county and the school could therefore access, at that time, workshops, masterclasses, annual concert performances and national and international competitions. However, we found that they were geared towards mainstream student abilities and the music specialists that visited our school could not seem to adapt to our students' levels of ability or understanding.

I was determined that our students should have the opportunity to have music delivered in a way that suited them, but the authority still insisted on deducting an SLA for music from the school but provided no music support from 2010. In 2010 I researched how I could provide therapeutic music for all students. I did not have the budget for a qualified Music Therapist; indeed, we were still paying the authority for a music service we did not receive. And then I found out about therapeutic music.

Staff training

I believe that it is a priority to give staff in a special school the appropriate training to meet the needs of the students and to understand the conditions students are diagnosed with. I would say that the professional development of staff is the key to a school's success. Not only does it give a headteacher confidence in the delivery of an appropriate curriculum, as well as the technological and therapeutic interventions, but it also gives the member of staff confidence and makes them feel valued.

Members of staff who had no experience of working with the students attending our school were given time out of class, on a rota basis, to study free online courses to equip them for working in a special school such as ours. One such free site is www.ComplexNeeds.org.uk, which has training materials for teachers and support staff of learners with severe, profound and complex learning difficulties. There are 16 modules and a study planner. You can download materials to work offline if you need to. A free online study site provided by the NHS is www.MindEd.org.uk, which supports the study of the health and well-being of students. The open university provides a free course on understanding autism and they also provide 900 free courses on their Open Learn site. There are other free online learning providers. Our school also signed up to the online training provided by Educare (part of the TES) for training in safeguarding and any latest government initiative such as radicalisation. There is a cost, but we found the material robust, engaging and easy to use. Staff in a special school also require training in managing behaviours and supporting students with medical needs and care needs. It has always been an argument for special school headteachers that governments should give special schools more training days. Staff training takes a huge chunk out of the budget in a special school and I continually chased extra funding and other ways of meeting the training needs of the staff. Staff in our school knew they would be supported in their professional development and were very keen to develop their skills to meet the needs of the students.

Therapeutic music

I was fortunate enough to have a teaching assistant who had studied music at university and was willing to do an online Therapist in Music course. There are such courses available online and they are very reasonably priced. On average, they require 150 hours of work and so the person must really want to do it and have the academic capabilities to do the course.

As a result of the teaching assistant undertaking the training, I was able to employ her as an unqualified teacher and she enjoyed the role of therapist in music so much that after two years she went back to university to undertake training as a teacher. As luck would have it, we had another teaching assistant with a degree who wanted to take on the role and she also did the online training. She decided to retire last year, and a male teaching assistant, also with a university degree, asked if he could do the online training. He job-shared with her until she retired fully in 2019. He then took on the role full time.

Music sessions took place individually, in pairs or small groups depending on the needs of the child. The students are able to find a safe place through the music to explore their feelings and to learn strategies for managing their own behaviour. We have used the therapy to support individuals who struggle with behaviour, and one particular student would modify her behaviour knowing that she had therapeutic music to look forward to at the end of each day. The therapist also led each term's music production and was in charge of music assessment for students throughout the school. The school has benefited hugely from having a therapist in music. It was the only way that we could afford it.

Both research and practice have demonstrated therapeutic music to be an effective means of reducing the anxieties and associated behaviours that result from emotional turmoil. This has been evident in the progress made by the students at Pen Coch who were identified as having behavioural difficulties.

I vividly recall a young boy aged nine joining us from mainstream. He had, supposedly, huge behavioural issues and the SEN advisor for the county felt that our school was his last hope. We found on his first visit to our school at the end of a summer term that he loved music and especially the keyboard, though he was unable to play a note. He joined our school in the autumn term and attended therapeutic music with Chris, our therapist in music. He did not have behaviour problems. He just could not do the work expected of him in a mainstream school. His excellent class teacher Pauline came to show me his writing that he had torn up in frustration on his first day with his new class. She was able to show him that it was just fine motor skills and she helped him to develop his computer skills to ease his frustration at not being able to produce what his mind wanted to. His favourite piece of music was from CBeebies and the *Night Garden* when it signalled time for toddlers to go to bed. The SEN advisor for the county and his parents attended our Christmas concert at the end of his first term. The advisor was visibly moved, and his parents cried as they watched him play that piece of music on the keyboard as baby Jesus was put in his crib to sleep.

We saw consistent improvements in behaviours through the use of therapeutic music in the ten years that I was headteacher at the school. Teachers reported that in some cases students' social skills improved over time. The therapists worked closely with the teachers and were able to tackle specific individual education plan (IEP) targets set by the teacher in a uniquely engaging environment.

Here is a link to the amazing Chris giving a therapeutic music session: https://youtu.be/x RGHMm3poMg?list=PL-a5MUplgl4nVMUEFGUGFg4jTxjvPyLur.

The course that those wonderful members of staff undertook introduced the participants to an understanding of music therapy, its history and what a therapist does. It also gave the person insight into its use for conditions such as autism, learning difficulties, mental health issues, anxiety, pain relief, dementia and depression. It provided evidence of its beneficial effects on sleep and behaviour. It introduced the person to the different kinds of music therapy and how to select appropriate music. It showed how flexibility is an important aspect of being a therapist and how to structure a session with an individual as well as group session. I was told by them all that it was a very thorough course. The most recent person to attend the course in 2020, Gavin, shared this with me:

> The course was a bit hit and miss as there were 3–4 units that really helped and had some good background information about the benefits of music therapy for children with autism. Other units were giving me the full history of music therapy and some were aimed at independent practitioners in psychiatric wards, for example, which were a bit of a slog. But I completed it and I am glad I did it.

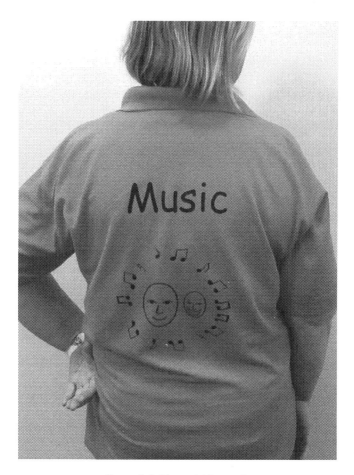

Figure 1.1 Therapist in music

This person has worked with students with special needs for a number of years and has a natural ability of gaining their trust and encouraging them to blossom. He wrote to me recently:

> I feel that it is going very well, thank you for the opportunity. I'm very happy within my role as it allows me to be creative, it challenges me and the response I get from children and staff is very positive, so I get a lot of satisfaction from the role.

Below is how he has developed the role:

> I completely emptied the music room, got rid of everything that wasn't necessary in the room and I have set up the Soundbeam within the room, so it is accessible to all pupils/staff, whenever they want to use it; that way, it doesn't get damaged going to each class.
> I have put all instruments together in their specific areas (drums all together, guitars all together, etc.) and I have used communication in print to label each area, so it is easier for

children to locate the instruments that a certain session is aimed at. The Skoog is also set up within the room, but I do take that out with me if I've planned it into a group session.

In the summer, I came up with a structure for group sessions that I stick to and it has been working very well.

I have written my own songs – a hello song, a how are you song and a goodbye song; the children will sing these back to me now/respond and it prompts communication in every session, regardless of behaviour, etc.; this is the bare minimum expectation I set.

I will always do a movement activity at the start of the session – be it 'head, shoulders, knees and toes' or something along those lines. That will be followed by a literacy/numeracy-based song where I play the guitar/sing the song and the children play percussion instruments along with me/sing the song/count along, etc. Then I'll have a focus activity for each lesson, which will involve a listening activity, exploration of an instrument, and explore a different type of dynamic from the group, be it tempo, rhythm, notation, etc. I also love storytelling through music and expression of emotions. The structure really helps the sessions as it allows for turn-taking, communication opportunities, teamwork and I can set realistic targets suitable for each child within that group. It also makes the children appreciate other abilities.

In the higher ability groups, I allow children to take over and compose their own pieces of music; once I've set the activity, I let them make their own decisions and this allows for discussion and self-evaluation opportunities. I've had several great opportunities since starting the role, most recently working alongside an author to bring his book to life when he visited the school, using music and sensory elements in the hall. It was fantastic as you can imagine!

If you or your school are interested, then follow the links below to check out course content before you choose whether the course meets your school's needs. It will be a continuous assessment course.

The course will usually take your staff member up to 150 hours to complete working from home. There is no time limit for completing these courses, it can be studied in their own time at their own pace. The course comes with a course assessment in the form of quizzes, written questions and short essays. Once the staff member has completed the course assessment, they email or post it back to the course organisers for marking, and the staff member will then receive feedback and certificates. As the school pays for the course the school should ask for a copy of the certificate once gained to share with the governors of the school.

Most courses are accredited by the CMA (Complementary Medical Association) but you would need to satisfy yourself of that beforehand. Below are two of the websites we used, and both courses cost well under £200. This is a cost-effective way of providing therapeutic music, but you must do your homework and you need to ensure that you have a suitable staff member in mind who is willing to put in the time to study. I tended to give a time limit of when I wanted it completed, and as the member of staff would have a salary increase once they received the certificate, they were more than happy to oblige.

- www.reed.co.uk/courses/music-therapy-course/80628
- www.centreofexcellence.com/shop/music-therapy-course

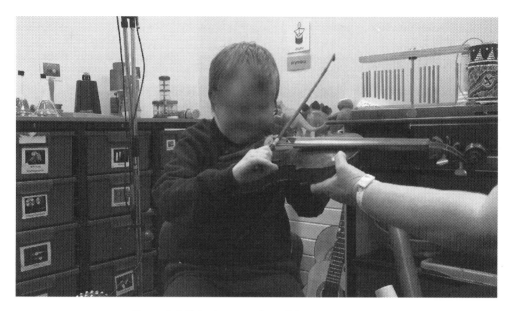

Figure 1.2 Enjoying a session of therapeutic music

No course can make you into a good therapist or teacher; only your dedication and commitment can do that. And I knew we had that with Gavin. I remember observing him delivering therapeutic music during our after-school club with an elderly client who had autism. It brought tears to my eyes. He really was that good. He ended the session by giving her a waltz around the room. She had found it so difficult to get up the courage to enter our building a year previously, and to see how far therapeutic music had taken her was wonderful.

If you do go down the road of training a member of your own staff, you can then decide if you can afford to employ them full time or part time or if you wish to have a job share. All of the therapists I employed had T-shirts displaying the therapy that they delivered as a visual reminder for students and visitors.

Here is a link to watch a therapist in music in action at Ysgol Pen Coch: https://www.youtube.com/watch?v=xRGHMm3poMg.

Outside agencies

Some schools invite outside agencies in to support the delivery of therapeutic music. Here you can see a video of the charity Jessie's Fund running a Soundtracks project with the Mabel Pritchard Community special school in 2020. The charity has been providing such support for over 25 years: https://youtu.be/rLgoT6YNy1Q. They also provide very resonably priced training, including CPD certificates.

Jessie's Fund can be contacted at:

15 Priory Street, York,
Y01 6ET, United Kingdom
Phone: (+44) 01904 658 189
E-mail: info@jessiesfund.org.uk

In 2002 parents of a child with autism set up the charity Music for Autism. This charity provides support to special schools as well as concerts specifically for those with autism. Go to www.musicforautism.org to find out more.

Soundabout Soundabout (Registered charity number 1103002) is a charity that uses music to empower and unlock the potential of people with severe and profound learning disabilities. Soundabout have their own TV channel and provide online sessions for you to join. Go to https://youtu.be/2TvmBbtABCE to see for yourself.

Music Making SENse is a team of professionals who work in partnership with special schools developing a bespoke music curriculum whilst supporting and mentoring both teachers and teaching assistants. To see them in action, go to https://www.musicmakingsense.com/.

YAMSEN: Specially Music, supported by the Heritage Lottery Fund, has created a set of free multisensory music and arts cross-curricular resources about the Leeds Liverpool Canal.

The pack includes:

* A teacher's book with clear instructions showing the activities for different levels of working
* A CD with the songs recorded as learning tracks and as singalong tracks
* An illustrated pupil's book which includes the song words, art and dance ideas

The resource pack is also available in hard copy via post. For books, please contact Leeds for Learning stating your school name and how many teacher's and pupil's books are needed.

PAMIS is an organisation in Scotland that works specifically with those with PMLD. I have been inspired by this organisation and what they do. One of their Music Therapists Fiona Sharp produces support material for those providing therapeutic music for students and adults with PMLD. If you visit www.pamis.org.uk you can find out more.

There are many exceptional Music Therapists providing support to schools, prisons, hospitals and communities. The Otakar Kraus Music Trust (OKMT) is based in the London Borough of Richmond and provides music therapy for people of all ages who have physical, psychological, learning, behavioural or emotional difficulties. They also introduced the first clinical music therapy into India. If you wish to find out more, go to www.okmtrust.org.uk/contact.

Of course music is therapeutic in many contexts and I remember taking a group of students with profound and multiple learning difficulties to Gloucester Cathedral to listen to a recital in 2002. The vaulted ceilings and beautiful surroundings added to the experience for the students. I know that many special schools take students to cathedrals and concerts as a regular occurrence. Everyone deserves music in their lives.

If you decide to set up a therapeutic music room, then you will need to do a risk assessment and provide health and safety guidance. A music room risk assessment is included in chapter 13 for you to copy. A therapeutic music report template is also available in chapter 13. Feel free to copy the health and safety guidance below.

Health and safety and the use of musical instruments in therapeutic music

- Staff members are responsible for their safety and the safety of their students.
- Ensure all musical equipment is regularly tested and examined.
- Ensure all instruments and equipment are cleaned after each use.
- You should be careful if lifting large instruments (e.g. xylophones, large drums) or the Soundbeam. Attend any training you can in safe moving and handling practice. Use trolleys/wheels wherever possible, allow enough time not to rush, and get help to move large items.
- Drums/tambourines – look out for splinters in wood, holes in skins (where small fingers could be trapped), sharp points (e.g. nails which hold jingles on tambourines can come loose or stick out), loose screws/tightening nuts which could come off and be swallowed, etc. Look out also for splinters on drum sticks (from being hit against the rim). Discard these.
- Sticks/beaters – the main danger here is loose heads which may come off and be swallowed – a particular risk with small beaters and small children. Remember that physically or neurologically disabled students or developmentally delayed students may be particularly vulnerable to accidental swallowing, or lack an effective gag reflex. Always check such beaters before use (pull hard!) or use sticks/hands.
- Resonance boards – place the boards so that there are no gaps in which fingers could be trapped. Remove shoes and socks if necessary. Socks can cause slipping on the board. Students with limited movement may need to keep shoes on so that their small movements create sound.
- Blowing instruments – these should not be used with students who are immuno-depressed, immune-suppressed or otherwise vulnerable to infection. Ensure sterile/anti-bacterial wipes are used after each use. Do not permit students to run with these in their mouths (danger of falling/choking).
- Ensure all broken instruments and equipment are repaired or destroyed and that damage is reported so that the school damage reporting procedure may be followed and a record kept.

To deliver music as a therapy requires an understanding of technological developments in music.

So what are these developments? We will look at these in the next chapter.

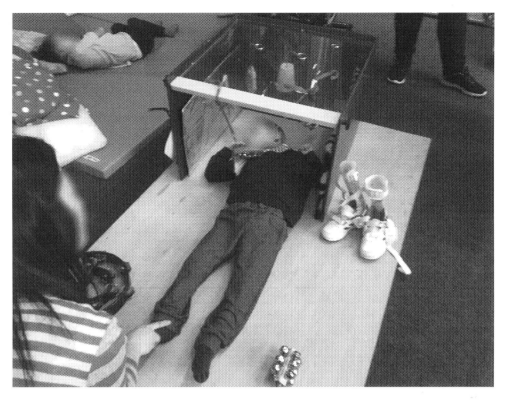

Figure 1.3 Using a resonance board

2 Music and technology for those with special needs

In this chapter I explore the innovative music hardware and software currently available to those working with students who have learning differences. I believe the Covid-19 pandemic has utterly changed an education system that was already losing its relevance. We have been teaching in a 19th century system using 20th century teaching methods with 21st century technologies available to us for a long time. There have been pockets of excellence where some schools have been taking full advantage of the technological advancements available, but often schools get caught up in a kind of hand-to-mouth existence where they cannot find time to explore and use all the new available technology. Added to that is the lack of training for teachers to use innovative technology. We are in the fourth industrial revolution and schools and universities are now being made to make full use of its technological advancements because of the pandemic. Governments around the world have, in recent years, spent millions on education reform. I believe that a new hybrid model of education will emerge from this pandemic just as the phoenix emerged from the ashes.

Initial training for teachers should include an understanding of how to use technology to its best advantage in schools, and, once qualified, teachers should expect their school to provide them with continued professional development in technological skills to keep pace with technological developments. In this technological age, all teachers should be technologically competent.

It is important for schools to prioritise the professional development of their staff and ensure that staff training in technology is continually updated because technology is advancing at an exponential rate. This is the age of technology and every member of staff working with students should be up to date with technological developments. The technological advancements in music for students with special needs over the last few years are fantastic. Staff in special schools need to be given time to be trained in these new music technologies.

If you work with students who have learning differences or physical disabilities, you will have come across the terms Alternative and Augmentative Communication (AAC) and Adaptive Music Technology (AMT). AAC is the use of communication methods to help them to write and speak. AMT is the adapted use of specialist music technology software and hardware to help them to take part in music.

Pioneering work in both these technologies is transforming the lives of students. When I was teaching students with learning differences in the 1990s, the best technology I could offer them was the opportunity to listen to music and to press a switch to turn it on/off. That being said, we did use music and technology to its full advantage to encourage communication for our students with PMLD. As far as assessment is concerned, it would be classed as the old P level 4 of cause and effect and would certainly be worthy of celebration as students with PMLD are often considered to remain at P levels 1–3 (see Section 20 of the Appendix).

In the 1990s we would give our teenage students with PMLD music from different popular artists to listen to and a connecting switch to turn the music back on or turn it off altogether. This helped us to discover who their favourite artists were. We were then able to inform their carers or parents for them to try outside of school so that the students could enjoy music of their choice rather than music imposed upon them. I remember being asked to visit a care home where one of our students resided to see how a care worker had copied our idea and had set up a music system in Matthew's room with switches for him to activate the music. It was really good, and we hoped that the care worker would share his knowledge with others at the home so that Matthew could continue to have that independence. We found that Johnathan, aged 14, got very excited and happy when he heard techno music, but at home parents played classical music. Because of our discovery they bought techno music for him to listen to in his room.

Machine learning today is able to look at patterns that we cannot see, in music, sound and images. Refik Anadol is able to use his talents in the field of technology to produce works of art using visual archives accompanied by sound archives put into a conscious latent space, and then regurgitate them into this world, spitting out visual and auditory memories that can then be projected onto buildings. It is data of music and sound made beautiful. To see a striking example of this, visit www.laphil.com/about/watch-and-listen/walt-disney-concert-hall-dreams-relive-the-epic-performance. This performance is available for students and their families to watch and schools need to be mindful of the access that students have to technology outside of school. Even if a teacher does not have the abilities of Refik Anadol, they can certainly share his work with students.

The technological revolution today not only allows students to listen to their favourite music with visual images, but they can also take part in that music just by using an iPad.

iPad apps

The iPad has an increasingly important role within mainstream and assistive music technology. Every day more music apps are added to the app store and it is well worth browsing to see if there is something new to use on your class.

Leicestershire Music provide a list of free music apps that are available on their site. To find out more, go to www.leicestershiremusichub.org.

Several apps exist which turn the iPad into a touch-sensitive synthesiser as well as a movement-to-audio converter. AUMI is one such app and it is free. Go to www.aumiapp.com to download it and learn how to use it. You can just go to the Apple store and download it for free, but the website gives you a lot of support while the app store does not. If you are into music apps, then it might be easy for you to use, but I found that I needed the help on the website and my music therapist friend also preferred downloading the free instruction manual from the website as it saved time. AUMI can be used by students with profound and multiple learning difficulties (PMLD) and those with severe learning difficulties (SLD), as well as more able students.

ThumbJam is not free and is available on the app store. However, it is an extremely popular music app with musicians. It has many useful tools and a large selection of factory pre-set samples. If you go to www.improviseapproach.com it will show you how to set up the app for use with students with severe, profound and complex needs.

Solfeigo.io is a web-based app for teaching popular music. It works with the interactive white board and students can access the app at home (https://solfeg.io/).

Beamz is a free-to-download iPad music app available from https://thebeamz.com. The website also provides training videos on how to use the app. It is built to support multiple access methods – switches and mouse alternatives, touch surfaces (screens and interactive boards), adapted keyboards and Eye Gaze.

Eye Harp is a free music app to be used specifically with the Eye Gaze. Go to http://theeyeharp.org/ for a free download and learn how to use it. It is a gaze-controlled digital musical instrument allowing those with profound physical disabilities the ability to learn to play music. Go to chapter 12 for a free Eye Gaze policy to download.

Bloom is a music app that is not free but is fairly cheap. A student needs to be able tap or drag a finger on the screen. This produces colourful visuals with background music. If the student takes their finger off, then the music stops. And so, they learn about cause and effect. A teacher told me that her students became calm and focused while using the app. It is easily available on the Apple app store; go to https://apps.apple.com/us/app/bloom/id292792586. A similar app, also not free, is Trope. Go to https://apps.apple.com/us/app/trope/id312164495 to download it.

The Skwitch Music app was designed to integrate Skwitch with the technology built into your iPhone. The app interacts with Skwitch and has in-app guides and videos to help you with getting started. Using patented magnetic sensing technology, it will turn the slightest touch on the button into expressive musical sound. It can be found on the Skoog site. Go to https://skoogmusic.com/skwitch/.

Sometimes we listen to a piece of music and cannot recall who wrote it or recorded it. Sometimes a student will be humming a tune that they like but cannot tell you the name of it. An app named *Shazam* can be downloaded onto an iPad or phone, and if you play a couple of seconds of the music or indeed hum the music as you tap on the Shazam logo, it will immediately tell you the name of that piece of music and who wrote it. Go to www.shazam.com/gb/apps to find out more.

Google has launched its 'Hum' feature where you can hum/whistle/sing into its search engine and it can recognise the tune. To get it working, open the latest version of the Google app or widget. Tap the microphone icon and say, 'What's this song?' Do your best attempt to hum/whistle/sing the tune to get a result.

As technology advances, new and improved versions of the above apps will be released and it is important that teachers keep abreast of these developments. We live in the technological age. All subjects, including music, can now be enhanced through the use of technology. Nowhere is this more important, to my mind, than in the field of special education. At last students get the opportunity to really participate in actually making music.

Soundbeam

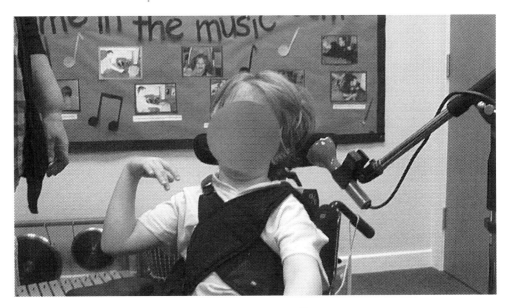

Figure 2.1 Using Soundbeam

There is a need for a brief introduction to Soundbeam so that anyone who has never used it or considered its use may be helped to decide on its use in their school or organisation. Choosing to fund a Soundbeam in a school is a commitment that needs to be agreed by all staff. The Soundbeam is an expensive and important set of equipment that should not be left in a cupboard because the only person who wanted it in the school has left the school.

I have used the Soundbeam in three special schools and I underwent Soundbeam training in the late 1990s. If your school is expecting all teachers to teach music to their class and have the opportunity of including the use of the Soundbeam in the lessons, then each teacher will need to be trained.

If your school has decided to nominate a single teacher or therapist to deliver Soundbeam to the students, then only that person needs to be trained. I would recommend that at least two members of staff are trained so that if the nominated person is absent or leaves the school the other person can take over. Students become reliant on a therapy or piece of technology. It is ignorance on our part to assume that it does not matter if it is no longer available to them. Soundbeam is continually updated and newer versions brought out regularly. It is always best to get the latest version and vital that training is undertaken, as it is a complex piece of equipment.

I would recommend regular updated training. Soundbeam.co.uk have a 'Soundability' residential course annually which is well worth attending if you want to see what other schools and organisations are managing to achieve with their Soundbeams and if you want support to use it to the best effect for your school or organisation. If you wish to, find out more at www.soundbeam. co.uk/soundability-all-info-and-form.

I have said many times that the training of staff and their continuous professional development is one of the most important parts of a school development plan, and I really do believe that. Even if you have to raise funds to do so, you need to ensure that your staff keep up to date with the latest available training. It gives them confidence in delivering their subject when they are on top of their game. I would indeed be worried if my staff did not wish to update their skills because this impacts on the students. Because of this technological age many students attending special schools are more savvy about technology and it is important that staff do not fall behind but continue to earn the respect of their students.

What is Soundbeam?

Soundbeam is a 'touch-free' device that uses sensor technology to translate body movement into music or sound. It gives students, regardless of their disability or impairment, the opportunity to play music. Soundbeam has pre-loaded sound sets that enable explorations of various genres and enables students to create their own compositions. The device is loaded with all sorts of different instruments that may well be inaccessible to them ordinarily. I have used the Soundbeam technology, when I was a teacher, to great effect and I have listened as a headteacher as students have used Soundbeam to create ghostly music for a Halloween disco or Christmas music for a pantomime. I have also attended a National Arts competition with students and our therapist in music as our students acted out Peter and the Wolf using the Soundbeam.

What are the benefits of Soundbeam?

Soundbeam allows users to form a musical language of their own or within a group. It is a great way for students to learn about cause and effect and intentionality. I have watched enthralled as a student has suddenly become aware that the slight movement of their head has caused the Soundbeam to activate music. It is magical to watch as the student eventually begins to compose their own music. This does take time and patience because a student can have erratic movement, and be able to activate the beam one minute only to take several attempts before it happens again. These sessions are best done one on one to begin with until the student has developed muscle memory. These compositions can be recorded and played back to a class so that the student achieves a sense of pride and achievement – but only if the student has communicated that they would like others to listen or watch their performance. Always bear in mind that just because a student has a label of PMLD, and you may think they do not understand social etiquette, they still warrant respect.

I have attended performances where groups of students have worked together to deliver the background music for Christmas concerts using the Soundbeam. They have orchestrated a piece of music between them. It has allowed everyone to take part, some of them pressing switches to activate music, thereby promoting inclusion. It has proved to be a stimulating and rewarding experience for them and, in my experience, parents love to see their children taking part.

Soundbeam requires a commitment from staff. Some schools prefer to use cheaper alternatives such as iPad apps. It is a decision senior management need to consider with as much professional advice as possible bearing in mind the size and context of the individual school. The Soundbeam is continually updated to keep abreast of technological innovations and I would always recommend getting the very latest version so that students have the very best opportunities to create music.

Skoog

Skoog is not a Swedish lager. It is a tactile musical instrument that allows users to compose and create sounds in a fun way that incorporates colour and a true sensory element to music-making. Using its tactile sensors, it can pick up on motion and movement and can translate them into sounds.

Skoog is a fully accessible piece of equipment that is perhaps less imposing than the Soundbeam. We bought the white version. The white surround is foam-like and pliable. Its sensitivity to touch is adjustable so that you should be able to activate its sensors just by placing your hand on the Skoog. You can interact with it by using any part of the body – touching, squashing, shaking, tapping with hand, foot, knee or chin.

To activate the Skoog, you just need to press the button at the base of the Skoog.

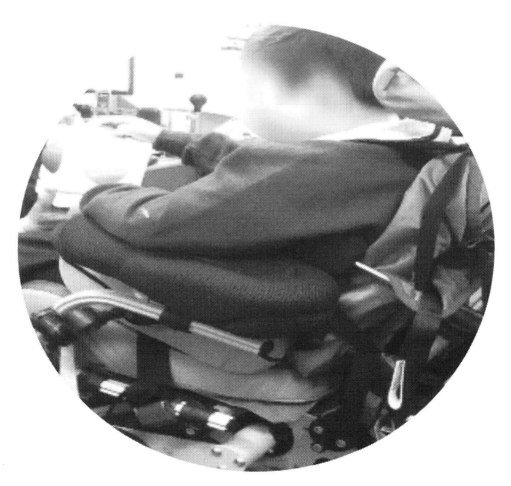

Figure 2.2 Using the Skoog to make music

* It helps to develop social skills
* It helps to develop communication.
* It improves concentration.
* It encourages participation.
* It encourages self-expression.
* It develops physical skills.
* It is accessible for all.

Make sure you learn how to use it properly before using it with students. The website has plenty of support and videos to show you how to use it. The site also provides lesson plans. Go to https://skoogmusic.com/support/.

For individuals: An individual is able to access the Skoog quite easily and in early sessions the Skoog app can integrate with your iTunes library or Spotify account so that they can use the Skoog to play along to any of the student's favourite music that they might usually listen to.

For groups: The Skoog can be used in group music sessions for students who perhaps would not be able to participate ordinarily, using traditional instruments. It allows inclusivity. You can use music apps such as Garageband with the Skoog and take part in an orchestra using it. As the Skoog is just a cube it is a quicker way of providing access to music-making than setting up the more complex Soundbeam.

Brainfingers®

Brainfingers® is a special headband fitted with switches that respond to minute facial movements and convert them to computer key commands and/or MIDI. Current development of Brainfingers® is looking at picking up the alpha and beta brainwaves (if you have used a neurofeedback machine you will see these brainwaves at work) so that musical events could be triggered just by thinking. Technology is so exciting.

Digital technology

Digital technology allows disabled people to be able to make music, and for non-disabled people to do it more easily. There are a number of music engineers and music technicians who have developed the use of assistive technology, who have adapted conventional instruments to be played more inclusively in new ways. The university of Huddersfield has an Adaptive Music Technology Research Group (AMTRG) which seeks to bring together universities, companies and schools to promote the wider adoption and development of this technology.

Tod Machover's work at MIT's media lab experiments with developing new technologies that encourage and enable people from all walks of life to create new music. He has given a TED Talk and was joined by Dan Ellsey, a man with cerebral palsy who had a piece of technology designed specifically for him and who performs an instrumental piece 'My Eagle Song'. With the right tools and technology everyone is capable of expressing themselves through music.

Tod Machover says, 'Everyone can experience music in a profound way. We just have to make different tools' (https://www.youtube.com/watch?v=Zj2QoLhfwew).

There are also charities that support people of all ages and a wide range of disabilities to play, learn and compose music independently. Drake Music Scotland is one of these. Beginning with a three-member group in 2012 and growing to a quartet in 2013 and ensemble in 2014, Drake Music Scotland launched Scotland's first disabled youth orchestra in 2016. With subsequent performances in Singapore and Norway, the orchestra has quickly become one of the world's leading disabled ensembles.

Drake Music Scotland created software for the inclusive music notation system Figurenotes in 2010 which over the decade has benefited more than 15,000 learners. Figurenotes is a simple coloured shape matching system which makes it easy to read music and learn to play instruments such as the keyboard and guitar. The software has won the Music Teacher UK 'Best Special Educational Needs Resource' award. Music Teacher UK also has its own free online resources to aid anyone wanting to learn music (www.musicteachers.co.uk/resources/funstuff).

In 2010, Drake Music Scotland launched a new partnership with Edinburgh College which has helped over 60 school leavers with learning difficulties gain accredited qualifications in Music Technology.

As well as using the well-known Soundbeam, Skoog and iPad, Drake Music also makes use of the Eye Gaze. The Eye Gaze is used in many special schools today and allows the student to use their eyes to communicate and even to play the keyboard.

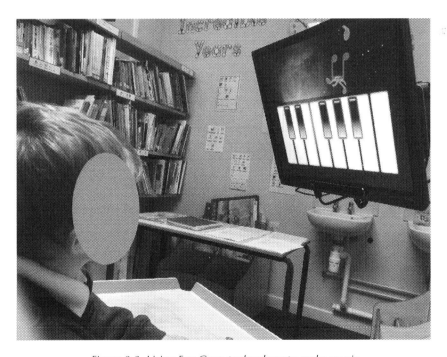

Figure 2.3 Using Eye Gaze technology to make music

To see one of our students playing the keyboard using Eye Gaze, go to https://youtu.be/06NE
v8faxKl?list=PL-a5MUplgl4kU9ANyKh_BpUoQ2G9lkcc4.

In 2019 Drake Music Scotland was the only UK organisation to use the Brainfingers® technology to enable people to make music. As mentioned earlier in the chapter, Brainfingers® consists of a headband fitted with sensors that read the brainwaves generated when the player chooses an option shown on the computer screen. For more information on the exciting use of technology made by Drake Music and to be able to see a student using the Eye Gaze to be part of an orchestra, go to https://drakemusicscotland.org/about/.

There are individual schools that excel in the use of assistive technology tools to make music more accessible and fun. Rawchestra formed by Melland High School Academy, a special school in Manchester, uses iPads, Soundbeams, switches, assistive apps and adapted musical instruments to produce concerts and performances. It often combines with another school on campus (Cedar Mount). If you want to get ideas on how you could do this and to see them in action, go to https://www.youtube.com/watch?v=Lk2Rbnw2jUY.

Specialist technology and online support

The Amber Trust has an online resource for teaching music to blind children called Amber Sound Touch. This site was launched by the Amber Trust charity and the ISM Trust. Both charities do an amazing amount of work. To see how this online resource works, go to https://youtu.be/-2TDYFjTofo.

Apollo Ensemble is a completely integrated AMT system developed by Mark Hildred at Apollo Creative. It comprises a wide range of switches and sensors which you can choose to suit people's abilities, plus a wireless PC interface and software which interprets the messages from those switches to convert into sounds.

E-Scape is a sequencer designed especially for disabled musicians and those with special needs. It has integrated facilities enabling total control from switches. It provides automated auditioning for editing 'by ear', and guidance through processes, and has enabled many people who could not use standard music software with a switch overlay to learn about and create music without help.

Music is a vibration (MIAV) was a collaboration between Sense artist Justin Wiggan and Tom Peelat working with emerging technology and traditional sources of music to enhance emotional health and well-being. The toolkit produced from this collaboration offers a range of inclusive musical activities, especially for students with complex disabilities. It is free and is available at www.sense.org.uk/music.

Musicca.com is a free-to-use, ad-free site created for students of all levels. All exercises are self- correcting, and designed to ensure the most effective learning pathway, whilst still being fun and easy to use. Prior musical knowledge is not essential. Go to www.musicca.com.

Charanga is music education technology, digital music programmes, partnerships, and training for teachers. It offers music teaching and learning, a curriculum with a library of resources, and its website will tell you that in 2020 it was used by 41,000 teachers in 62 countries, so is worth taking a look at. It also has a home learning section called Yumu. Go to https://charanga.com to find out more, or go to https://youtu.be/88wylwjCNBk to see SEND technology in action.

The University of the Arts London (UAL) Creative Computing Institute (CCI) runs online after-school clubs on YouTube. 'How to make sounds with machine learning' is one of their 2020 videos that you can adapt to use with your students. Go to https://www.youtube.com/watch?v=oP_wx309asc. YouTube itself is highly popular with students. I recall one of our students with severe behaviour issues would calm down when listening to specific Turkish music on YouTube. His home language was Turkish.

Some schools have their own sound systems for students to listen to music. We had sound systems throughout the school, and this was immensely popular during special occasions such as Christmas.

It was also ideal for playing specific transitional music at certain times of the day. Let us look next at how schools can and do use music at times of transition.

3 Transitional music

If you have had babies in your family, you will have noticed that they recognise familiar tunes in a programme that you might watch regularly. I recall my ten-month-old daughter turning her head in recognition to the introductory music for the nightly six o'clock news programme.

If I were assessing her, I would say she was reacting to a familiar piece of music. She was meeting the criteria for R2 in the Sounds of Intent (SOI) framework.

We know that students with SLD and sometimes PMLD are able to show this emerging awareness of sound and so it makes sense to capitalise on this fact and use regular specific sounds/songs/musical interludes to signify specific times of the day. Music can provide order and pattern as well as a cue for what is coming next. This can allay the fear, flight or freeze reaction that could otherwise occur.

This is something that special schools have been doing for years. However, it is important that the same music/sound/song is used throughout the school and not changed when students move class, as it can take a good while for the student to adapt to a different piece of music, depending on their cognitive ability. It is useful to have a transitional music policy so that all staff realise its importance.

It is such an important aspect of a special school that it warrants a discussion in a whole school staff meeting and should be on the agenda of regular school department meetings to ensure that all staff understand its importance and are fully on board with its use and choices of music.

If, for instance, it has been decided to use Armand Marsick's La Source, Op. 12 (1912) on a student's iPad to signify it's time for hydrotherapy, then that should be agreed by the manager of the pool, it should be shared with senior management, and it should not be changed on a whim. It should become meaningful to students. If the student's reaction to that piece of music is monitored, it may show progression so this should be recognised by staff and shared with parents, as any progress, no matter how small, is significant. It can also be part of the student's assessment for music.

Transition times can include the introduction to the day. Often students gather together, and songs are sung to greet the day and introduce each student to the class. The repetition of this activity every day can settle students. Some classes may have a specific song for each student. If the song has proved effective, then it should be shared with other class teachers so that it can continue to be used. There is absolutely no point in reinventing the wheel.

Observation and assessment

It is useful to keep an assessment of a student's recognition and response to transition times. Does the student only respond to a particular piece of music? Does the student only react to a song, Stjepan Hauser on the cello, or the sound of a gong? Is it the vibrational sound that affects them? Does the student respond to every transitional sound, and if so how? Do they show happiness or anxiety? This is what teaching and assessment in a special school is all about. If we find out what kind of music, sound or vibration gets a reaction, we can then work with that to enable progress.

Sometimes we need to take a step back from assessing every lesson that the student is present in and instead observe them at transition times. Often, we use objects of reference to show a student where they are going to next, when quite often music will have more of an impact.

It is obvious that you would not wish to overload the day with musical transitions, and so a transition to maybe outdoor play would involve the right attire and a visual sign showing how many students can access that activity. I have noticed in my many classroom observations over the years as a special school headteacher, school advisor and as a school inspector that classes responded more quickly to directives issued through music/sound/song than directives given verbally.

Transition times can also include transferring from a wheelchair to a bed or a toilet seat, or assisting in the dressing process, as these can be major events for a child with PMLD. Changes of position are in themselves valuable learning experiences for the student who will need to undertake these transitions many times during their lifetime. To attempt to reduce that time can lead to a lack of care and respect for the student and so it can be useful to have a particular song or piece of music to accompany that transition. As that particular song or piece of music has a specified time span, then it allows for a safe unrushed experience. Because these experiences happen at home, too, or in a care environment, all parties should be informed of the music/sound/vibration used so that the student has more opportunities to use the reinforcer and so that the activity becomes easier for everyone involved.

It is important that a transitional music policy is adopted, agreed and adhered to by all members of staff and shared with families and carers. You may wish to copy and adapt the Transitional Music Policy which can be found in the Resources section of chapter 13.

In chapter 4 we will look at how singing and signing contribute to the curriculum of a special school.

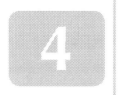

4   **Singing and signing**

Singing

If you go into any sing and sign session in a special school, you will hear a lot of sound. The voices are not always as harmonic as you might wish but they are enthusiastic. Yet if you think about it, when those of us who can speak put some earphones in and sing along to a song we like, it does not always sound as great to the uninvited audience. I wear headphones and carry my iPod in my pocket when I mow the lawn. I sing along to my playlist and get some strange looks from neighbours. Karaoke machines have been popular for some years now and we all think we sound better than we may actually sound to others when using the karaoke machine.

I remember when I was deputy head of an 11–19 special school in Herefordshire. We decided, as staff, that we would enter the local pub's karaoke competition. In the staffroom we suggested we dress up as the characters we were portraying, as each class were pretending to be a popular group. Our class were going to be the Beatles, so we raided charity shops and made face masks. On the night of the karaoke competition we all arrived at the pub. Our class were the only staff who dressed up and so we felt a bit foolish, but undeterred we got on stage and performed. I had altered the lyrics to 'Penny Lane' to fit in with the names and events of our school's respite centre. Obviously, in hindsight, it made no sense whatsoever to the audience that evening. The organisers of the karaoke night paid us £10 to get off the stage. I think we were hogging it a bit. A staff member took a video of the evening. When he played it back, we saw how dreadful we were, but we had enjoyed the evening and the camaraderie was great. We went on to perform it in school for the staff of the respite centre. The students in my class, all with PMLD, also took part in the assembly – as Beatles fans. By the way, even though I may not be very good at karaoke singing, I have found karaoke itself a great success for some of the students in my schools.

Mothers sing to soothe their babies to sleep. Lullabies can be found in every culture and every language. Parental songs arguably provide the most salient musical experiences in early life (Cirelli et al. 2019). Singing is naturally therapeutic, whether we are listening or doing the singing. It lifts our mood, releases dopamine and opens up many networks in the brain. We know that singing can improve breathing, posture, muscle tension and the reduction of respiratory symptoms

(Stacy et al. 2002). When members of a choir get together, they do more than sing together; they tend to breathe in harmony, too, and this can lead to stress reduction (Vickhoff et al. 2013). In 2020 Kate Corbett Winder writes in the *Guardian* of how she overcame panic attacks and depression by joining a choir (Winder 2020).

It goes without saying that more time is needed when teaching singing to students with learning difficulties, as you need to give them time to process the information and respond before moving on. Yet the great thing about singing is that you get the opportunity for repetition of skills learning without the monotony. Those of our students who can sing or sign easily learn the days of the week song and so can learn the order of the days of the week without realising they have done so.

When I was an assistant headteacher on the Channel Islands we had a weekly singing lesson on a Friday afternoon where all the children got together in the hall and the music teacher played the piano, instruments were handed out and we had a really good sing-song. The songs were highly appropriate for use in the classroom curriculum, including national songs, cultural and historical songs, popular songs, folk songs, etc. These songs were part of a potentially rich musical experience for the children and enhanced inclusion in the school. There was a great feeling of unity and a lovely way to end the week.

Some of our students in special schools have melodic singing voices and we have held special schools concerts at the beautiful St Asaph Cathedral in North Wales where students from Ysgol Plas Brodyffryn entertained us with their amazing singing. Ysgol Plas Brondyffryn is the regional centre for autism education. Sometimes I have watched their students with autism enjoy performing with their eyes closed or with their back to the audience. Other students with autism I have seen lose themselves in the performance and this allows them to ignore the audience so that they do not get stressed.

To watch an equally amazing special school sing "Hallelujah", go to https://youtu.be/boTn netaoJ8. The soloist has autism and ADHD.

Signing

In all the schools that I have worked in, inclusion has been developed because of the use of signing. From performing singing and signing at Gloucester Cathedral with students who attend both mainstream and special schools to performing at the North Wales special schools concerts; from competing in the North Wales choir competition to performing at old people's homes in Flint, with students from our adjoining mainstream school; singing and signing has been one of our most inclusive subjects.

In the North Wales choir competition, we were the only competitors not just singing but singing and signing. Our choir was made up of staff and students from both a special and a mainstream school. Although we did not win, we won a commendation. The students from both schools were delighted.

Many students in special schools love to sing but have difficulty forming some of the words. Students are encouraged in speech through learning sign language. Some students remain unable to speak but love to be part of a singing session and some are able to learn signs. A sing and sign session allows most students to take part. Sometimes being part of a choir and feeling the energy it produces is enough for some students who may appear to contribute little but benefit hugely. Learning sign language through singing is the easiest way, as it's repetitive, simple, slow and focuses on the language students need. Some students who cannot sign due to their impairments still wish to be part of the sing and sign group and this should be allowed if they are gaining something from the experience. If the experience is upsetting for a student, they will soon let you know.

Here you can see some of our students singing and signing the Lord's Prayer: https://youtu.be/bDeMRIJyFUg.

Signing is designed to be used either to enable the deaf community to communicate or to support spoken language and to help hearing people with SEN or with speech/language difficulties to communicate. The United Nations (UN) international day of sign languages is on 23 September every year.

British Sign Language (BSL)

British Sign Language (BSL) was recognised by the UK government as an official minority language in 2003. BSL was first used in a school in 1760 at Thomas Braidwood's academy for the deaf, so recognition has taken almost 250 years. It is now widely used, and my niece attends many music festivals with her boyfriend, who is deaf, and BSL interpreters accompany the performers.

BSL is a visual gesture language with its own structure and grammar, hand signs, body language, facial expressions and lip patterns. It is constantly evolving. I have only ever used it with deaf students.

Out of the Ark Music (outoftheark.co.uk) have worked with BSL specialists to produce instructional signing videos from their popular song collections: www.outoftheark.co.uk/video/signing/.

Sign Supported English (SSE)

Sign Supported English (SSE) uses the same signs as BSL but in the same order as spoken English. SSE is used to support spoken English.

Sign language is not universal. Music *is* a universal language, though, so singing and signing is immensely popular, as can be seen in these videos on YouTube. This particular group of signers use SSE and have appeared on the TV programme 'Britain's Got Talent'. The group are called Signalong with Us and also have their own website (www.signalongwithus.co.uk/) and YouTube channel (www.youtube.com/channel/UCKjnLaeAZiLeZpz6eDFPMrw).

Makaton and Signalong are much more recent methods of signing. It will depend on which local authority you work in as to whether Makaton or Signalong is used in your school, and you will need to use the preferred method for that authority. I have worked in different authorities throughout my career and have used both. Signalong and Makaton are both multi-modal signing programmes, combining signs from BSL, speech and symbols, and are designed to support those who have language and communication difficulties. The main difference is the method used to teach the programmes. Signalong has a larger sign vocabulary.

Makaton

Makaton was developed in the 1970s by speech therapists Margaret Walker MBE, Kathy Johnson and Tony Cornforth, and the term Makaton was created from combining the first syllables of each of their names.

To learn Makaton, you need to undertake training from a Makaton tutor. Many special schools have several staff trained as Makaton tutors. If you just wish to learn a few signs or try out Makaton, then head to their YouTube site for some free training: www.youtube.com/user/makaton charity.

In schools where I had Makaton tutors, they would start the whole school staff meetings with relevant, new or refresher signs for staff. They would display a weekly relevant sign in the corridors and would hold weekly meetings before school for staff requiring support and hold regular signing sessions throughout the week for students. They often led the sing and sign sessions. Makaton tutors have an important role in a special school, as they often lead the communication support which is a big part of any special school.

Mr Tumble, who appears on BBC CBeebies, is played by Justin Fletcher and he uses Makaton throughout his programmes. He is extremely popular with children. At the different schools I led, I purchased his DVDs and staff downloaded his YouTube videos to stimulate students' communication during indoor playtimes. One of our students was chosen to appear in one of his TV programmes. If you have not yet come across Mr Tumble, then a visit to see him in action is essential: www.bbc.co.uk/cbeebies/shows/something-special?%252523.

SingingHandsUK was formed by Makaton tutors Suzanne and Tracy. SingingHandsUK performed for us at one of our summer fayres at Ysgol Pen Coch and was hugely popular. SingingHandsUK has a YouTube channel showing nursery rhymes, pop songs and stories. Go to www.youtube.com/user/SingingHandsUK.

Total Communication is an approach that was widely used in Gloucestershire when I worked there as deputy head of a special school. It aims to make use of oral, signs, gestures, touch, eye pointing, auditory, written words and visual symbols and pictures depending on the needs of the student. Sometimes it can also mean communicating through dance or the arts. A very thorough introduction to signing can be found on their website: www.Totalcommunication.org.uk.

Signalong

Signalong was first devised as a resource that would be self-explanatory and accessible, offering a large library of over 9,000 signs giving a wide vocabulary. Once the methodology is understood, the clear line drawings in the manuals are easy to understand and I preferred using Signalong myself because of this.

At the special school where we used Signalong, the Speech and Language Therapists were very keen on the method and Signalong DVDs were developed with staff at the school teaching signs and songs.

I liked the fact that I could purchase Signalong books and learn the signs easily for myself. Although training is not required in the same way that Makaton is, training was set up in 1992 because of popular demand. Unlike British Sign Language training or that provided by some other organisations, Signalong training focuses on developing communication skills rather than teaching blocks of signs, many of which will be quickly forgotten through lack of use. To find out more, go to https://signalong.org.uk/. Signalong also has a YouTube channel with many rhymes and songs to learn: https://youtu.be/KuVlh_iXHbA.

DPAN

As you can see, there is no universal sign language. In fact, there are currently, according to Ethnologue.com, 144 sign languages in use, but another could be added to the list tomorrow, as manual signing differs geographically. Region and culture also play a large part in these differences.

In the same way that spoken languages change from country to country, so do sign languages. In the USA, for instance, American Sign Language (ASL) is used, and also Pidgin Signed English (PSE) which is the most common sign language used in the USA taken from ASL. Music is a universal language, though, and so singing and signing is immensely popular.

The Deaf Professional Arts network (DPAN) is an American non-profit organisation set up to promote music culture for the deaf and hard of hearing. Since 2006 it has its own YouTube channel for music videos utilising ASL. The music videos are for all of the latest popular songs. DPAN is well known by the Deaf/Hard of Hearing community in America. DPAN has managed to encourage the learning of ASL in schools across America because of its sign language TV channel. Although sign language is used in its videos, the videos are also captioned with written English to appeal to everyone. To find out more, go to https://www.bing.com/videos/search?q=Dpan+YouTube&FORM=RESTAB.

Singing and signing support

Soundabout was launched in 1995 in Oxford with the aim of empowering school staff working with children and young people with special needs to make music interactively with their students with severe and complex disabilities. In December 1997 Soundabout was officially founded as an independent charity that has pioneered the use of music, rhythm and sound to give disabled children and adults a voice, a way to express themselves and be listened to. They provide training programmes to schools. Go to https://youtu.be/klEJp2FwWTM to see how they managed to continue singing during the Covid-19 lockdown.

Another popular YouTube channel is the Big Top multi-sensory music workshop which includes signing, use of Makaton symbols, singing and instruments, with lots of themes to choose from.

It is highly recommended for use in school or at home. Go to www.youtube.com/channel/UCyXShtCdi0nZ-DrJbUUIFvQ/videos.

Shabang! Inclusive Learning is another fun YouTube channel that entertains with Makaton signing, singing, drama and sensory learning. For an example, go to www.youtube.com/watch?v=qEtkwCOs_sA.

Helping students to communicate is an important aspect of special schools, but it is also important for students to be in the right frame of mind to want to communicate. In chapter 5 we will look at how special schools use music to provide different ways to help students be in the right frame of mind to learn.

5 Meditation and mindfulness

Sir Thomas Beecham, the renowned conductor, once said, 'The function of music is to release us from the tyranny of conscious thought' (Beecham 1978).

Mindfulness involves training our attention to experience the present moment, and it could be argued that students with severe or profound learning difficulties are always in the present moment. They do not appear to be constantly bothered by contents of consciousness. They are present but not constantly thinking. Eckhart Tolle (2009) would call it essence identity and the transcendent dimension of who you are. One only needs to observe a student with PMLD gazing at the leaves of a tree as they shimmer and flutter in the sunlit breeze to remember that sometimes being present is enough.

Looking after the mind is as important as looking after the body. It is just as important for students with autism, ADHD and a host of other learning differences, and so it becomes an essential part of the special school curriculum. This can be supported through the different therapies shown in this book which are delivered by many special schools already.

Mindfulness is on the curriculum of some mainstream schools and I would argue that a certain level of cognitive ability is needed for students to be able to understand the teaching of mindfulness as opposed to the experience of mindfulness. Professor Mark Williams, former director of the Oxford Mindfulness Centre, says that mindfulness means knowing directly what is going on inside and outside ourselves. Mindfulness involves paying close attention to whatever you are doing in the present moment – playing an instrument, listening to a piece of music or focusing on a whole song as it is sung. Mindfulness begins with paying attention to breathing in order to focus on the here and now. It can train students with autism or ADHD to give enough distance from disturbing thoughts and emotions to be able to observe them instead of reacting to them. Students who practise mindfulness regularly can acquire a sense of self-control and can find it empowering, helping them to avoid clashes with other students. Please see chapter 13 for a meditation and mindfulness policy you may wish to adapt and copy.

Autsit.net is one of the many websites devoted to promoting mindfulness and meditation for people on the neurodiversity spectrum. Meditation can help to lower stress levels and reduce brain chatter, and this is particularly useful for students with autism or ADHD.

There are now courses available for training staff in mindfulness. There is also the Mindfulness in Schools Project (MiSP). Once you have developed a regular mindfulness practice according to its dictates, you are ready to train to teach the programmes yourself. Smiling Mind is used extensively in Australia, and some schools in the UK use it, too. If you wish to find out more, go to www.smilingmind.com.au/education.

Mindfulness can be achieved through meditation. There are some famous meditation gurus, such as Joe Dispenz, who give guided meditation advice on YouTube. The only problem with YouTube is that adverts interrupt the meditation, so if you wish to try out a free app with 80,000 free guided meditations, music tracks that display how long the music lasts, plus guidance on meditation from 8,000 teachers, then the free app InsightTimer might be what you want. Go to www.insightimer.com. You should recognise it by its singing bowl logo. YouTube has many videos to support meditation with students. Here is one to try: https://youtu.be/9CdPQ7X1MzU.

Frequencies of sound

It is now widely known that there are specific frequencies of sound that have a healing effect on the human body. Two of the most widely used are 528 Hz (known as the miracle tone and often associated with DNA repair) and 432 Hz. If you go to YouTube and search for those frequencies, you will find a large amount of meditative music at those frequencies to listen to and to use in your classroom or in your therapy room. There are also many to be found on InsightTimer. Here is a YouTube channel for those particularly popular frequencies, but many more can be found by searching for 'spirit tribe awakening': https://www.youtube.com/watch?v=cXQ8y-1ddcA&list=PLQV40q_WSGWd02L1oQtkXKowmOiZndz13.

Binaural beats

Binaural beats have been used as a stimulus for inducing meditative states with some success (Jirakittayakorn and Wongsawat 2017). There are many research articles backing up the use of binaural beats to reduce anxiety. Reference can be found in the bibliography section of this book, including a link to the Robert Munroe institute for free binaural meditations and more information about binaural beats.

Binaural beats (from Latin 'with both ears') are like optical illusions for sounds. When your left ear hears a slightly different tone from your right ear, you perceive a beat that does not present in the music you listen to. To listen to binaural beats, a student will need a pair of stereo headphones and an MP3 player or another music system. There are no known side effects to listening to binaural beats, but make sure that the sound level coming through the headphones is not set too high. Lengthy exposure to sounds at or above 85 decibels can cause hearing loss over time.

Binaural beat technology could be a problem if the student has epilepsy, so the parents should speak to their doctor before trying it. If you are unsure for any reason, then check first with a doctor. I would always give parents/carers a consent form to complete before allowing any student to undertake any therapeutic intervention, and would ensure copies of their consent were stored safely. For an alternative website where you can find out more or purchase binaural beats downloads, go to www.binauralbeatsmeditation.com. InsightTimer also has a section of binaural beats meditation to use for free.

YouTube is also awash with binaural beats videos for all kinds of health benefits. These also have some great stimulating visuals for those who need help focusing (but bear in mind YouTube interrupts your meditation with adverts). It goes without saying that you will not get the intended benefits if you listen to those videos without earphones.

Surround sound

It is possible nowadays to give students an 8D audio experience. It is a very realistic experience and care must be taken as some of the sounds could be sounds that students are hypersensitive to. The final chapter in this book covers the topic of hypersensitivity to sound in more detail. To understand what I mean about 8-dimensional sounds, you may wish to listen to an explanation for yourself and would certainly need to before introducing 8-dimensional sounds to students. Here is a link to an understanding of 8D sound: https://youtu.be/zhqbXjQ8IP0.

Some people find that 8D sound can induce trance-like states. Videos of 8D sound are available on YouTube.

Sound bath

I have observed success for students using focused meditation with PMLD and SLD where music is used in meditation. Focused meditation can be accomplished using a sound bath where vibration can also be felt through specific meditative music. Deaf students can benefit, as the resonance of the tuning fork, gong or drum will travel through the body just as it does for a hearing person and can be felt as a vibration. I was able to observe a successful sound bath in action for students with PMLD when I supported a special school in Peterborough in 2019.

The concept of sound baths originated in Tibet some 2,000 years ago. Most sound baths take place in a room with other people, but some special schools can offer one-on-one experiences if they have the space. During a sound bath students can lie down or sit in chairs. The room is often darkened to calm students and heighten other senses. Instruments can be played from one place, though sometimes the instruments are brought around the room and sometimes played over the student's body. Students are free to relax and drift off where the sound takes them.

A sound bath focuses on bathing the students in the relaxing, meditative noise of sound waves from crystal bowls, gongs, drums, tuning forks or other instruments. The sound therapist will encourage students to relax before starting to play. The sounds will start off softly to ease the student in, but will get progressively louder (the volume never becomes unbearable as the sounds are played therapeutically). The playing technique can change frequently so there is no fixed rhythm. Instead of the noise giving students a headache, sound baths have the clever ability to soothe the mind. In general students should feel very calm and relaxed after a sound bath. However, on occasion, students have been known to be very emotional once the sessions are over. At the end of a sound bath there should a period of silence followed by advice and support by the sound therapist to the student or teaching assistant accompanying the student.

Holistic sound therapy session in Ysgol Y Deri

Cheryl Galea is the Holistic Sound Practitioner for Ysgol Y Deri. Ysgol Y Deri is currently the largest special school in Great Britain. She told me:

The aim within the therapy room is for our pupils to be relaxed and happy. Essential oils are used before the session has started.

Lighting plays a big part in our sound therapy session with different coloured material, as some pupils are drawn to different materials placed around the therapy room; visualisation and colour breathing are a place to start the sound therapy session.

The therapy room:

* For pupils to be relaxed and happy
* Essential oils
* Lighting from overhead lighting around the room
* Low therapy beds with beautiful soft covers and pillows
* Colour therapy breathing through the chakras

Visualisation, breath, coloured materials sound therapy session:

We start the sound therapy session with breathing up through our nose and out through our mouths, working with colours from our chakras listed below, i.e. the Crown chakra, and the colour purple for two breaths. We work with the breath and visualisation.

The first chakra is the colour purple; we imagine a cloud of purple mist or a cloud just in front of your face; imagine breathing this mist up through your nose and out through your mouth with the colour purple (×2 breaths for each chakra). Repeating each chakra and its colour, each chakra has its own note as well and plays a big part in which instruments we use: hand bells and symbols, noted hand chimes, chimes and noted bells. The chakra notes support our health and well-being.

Chakra colours:

* Crown – purple
* Forehead – indigo
* Throat – light blue
* Heart – pink or green
* Solar plexus – yellow
* Sacral chakra – orange
* Root chakra – red

Notes of the chakras:

* Crown – (A)
* Forehead – (B)
* Throat – (A)

* Heart – (F)
* Solar plexus – (E)
* Sacral chakra – (D)
* Root chakra – (C)

Vibrational instruments:

These beautiful vibrational instruments are toned. Some have one tone while others have multiple tones, i.e. the gong and singing bowls. Each tone matches a chakra, and supports our well-being and health. At some points on the body we can find blockages, where our chakras are blocked through trauma or health issues. Using toned vibrational instruments from the list below, we can release blockages held in the aura or energy field (biofield) that surrounds us:

* Bells and chimes
* Noted hand bells
* Noted hand chimes
* Rain stick
* Ocean drum
* Singing bowls
* Gongs
* Circular drum
* Noted xylophone
* Noted drum

Notes, tones and overtones vibrate around the room as each pupil sits or lies down, changing the patterns of their brain waves from alpha to gamma waves just before we go to sleep and dream. A relaxed calm feeling of warmth and happiness brings us to a point in meditation.

Here we can talk/sing about our feeling by voicing our own sounds; we chant or tone through the use of our voice. Our bodies feel the vibration of individual sounds made by each pupil, i.e. 'Om' ×3 is great fun. We alter our brain waves through vibrational instruments and musical notes and tones.

Brain waves:

* Alpha
* Beta
* Theta
* Gamma

Concluding vibrations and sounds from vibrational instruments play a big part in how we let go of our emotions.

Holistic sound therapy has changed pupils' behaviours and as an intervention clears and grounds their personalities, supporting more positive outcomes in life; with time, holistic sound therapy can change the future of our health and well-being. We can create better health and knowledge about our personal patterns and behaviours through vibrational instruments, musical notes and tones, using the breath, visualisation, colour with essential oils and meditation. And this creates positive outcomes for more mindfulness in our own lives.

Qui-Gong

Qui-Gong is an ancient Chinese practice based on meditative movement that aims to bring the body into balance and often incorporates healing sounds for specific organs in the body. Sometimes you will be expected to repeat the sounds like a mantra. InsightTimer has guided Qui-Gong available on its site. YouTube also has many of these videos if you feel your students would benefit. Here is one of them: https://youtu.be/FltV3zCAFdw.

Reflexology

Some special schools are lucky enough to offer reflexology to their students. Again, this is done as a focused meditation with both music and touch involved. This certainly can help with mindfulness and meditation, and if you follow the link you can see a student at Ysgol Pen Coch visibly relax whilst listening to calming music and receiving reflexology: www.youtube.com/watch?v=NKpZ6Ci2ujl.

When choosing a piece of music to play during your delivery of any therapy, it is useful to choose a composer that you enjoy listening to, as you will be listening to it a lot. Sometimes a

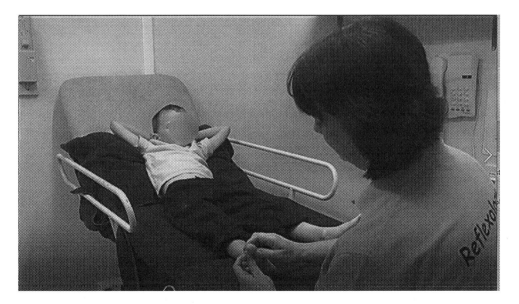

Figure 5.1 Reflexology and music meditation

student does not like a particular piece of music, so ensure you have some alternatives. Try and ensure that you present an entire piece of music and not merely a snatch of music. Tell the student the name of the composer and the name of the piece of music. Play that same piece of music, introducing it in the same way every time you deliver the therapy, unless the student communicates that they want a different piece of music. If they do want a different piece it is still important to let the student know the name of the piece and who composed it. You are giving both the student and the person who composed the music respect. If you have a picture of the composer, you might show it to the student.

Reflexology is the practice of applying pressure to and massaging certain areas of the feet. The aim is to encourage a healing effect on other areas of the body, including organs, glands and muscles, and improve general health and well-being. It is also sometimes referred to as 'zone therapy'. The length of the sessions depends on the needs/tolerance of the student. The relaxing effect of reflexology will be felt after the first session, but noticing benefits on other parts of the body may take longer.

It is possible to use reflexology as a form of meditative relaxation, rather than treating anything specific, in the way massage is used to relax. Reflexology is just one of the many alternative therapies currently unregulated in the UK. This means that there are no laws which state and detail the qualifications and level of experience someone must have in order to practise as a reflexologist.

Despite this there are a number of professional associations with whom practitioners can choose to register and become accredited. At Ysgol Pen Coch we had a member of staff with an accredited qualification in reflexology that the school financed. She was also a qualified aromatherapist. We used aromatherapy throughout the school.

Yoga

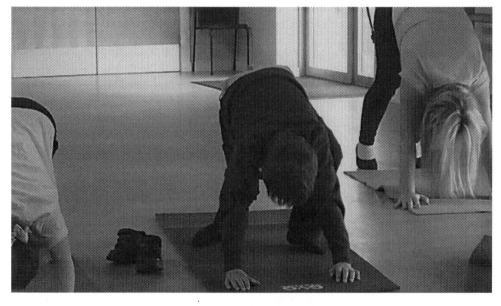

Figure 5.2 Yoga with music meditation

Another way of using focused meditation is through yoga with music.

In 2012 at Ysgol Pen Coch we investigated whether yoga to music would be a useful addition to the therapies we provided for our students:

- According to neuroscience our sense of who we are is anchored in our connections with our own body.
- All yoga programmes are made up of postures and stretches (*asanas*), and breathing (*pranayama*) and meditation.
- A significant proportion of our students were not aware of their breath, so learning to focus on breathing in and out and to count their breaths would help them get in touch with their bodies whilst reinforcing their number skills.
- Our emphasis was not on getting poses accurate but on helping students notice which muscles were active at different times.
- The sequences were designed to create a rhythm between tension and relaxation which we hoped would help them in their daily lives.
- Most of our students could not understand what was going on in their bodies. They were unable to tell anyone whether they felt physically unwell. They could not tell us what made them feel better or worse.
- Yoga can help those with autism to begin to appreciate sensory experiences. Cultivating sensory awareness is particularly important for students with autism so that they learn to anticipate and act on the ordinary demands of their body.
- Sometimes children with autism find it hard to tolerate their own sensations. In yoga, they learn to focus their attention on their own breathing and on their sensations moment to moment. Yoga therefore helped our students with autism to pay attention to how their actions make them feel. Staff volunteered to attend yoga classes and training sessions in their own time. It was unanimously agreed that Yoga would benefit the pupils. There are many Yoga programmes online available for schools to follow nowadays.

The programme that classes chose to follow at Ysgol Pen Coch was the Cosmic Kids programme, which is easily available for free on YouTube: www.youtube.com/user/CosmicKidsYoga.

For those of you who would prefer to use Qui-Gong with your students instead, then there is a routine available for children on YouTube. Go to https://youtu.be/eAQzFqdc7Hs.

Art, colour and meditation

Sometimes it is useful in focused meditation to focus on a piece of art. Dr Masaru Emoto produced meditation CDs to accompany his book *Water Crystal Healing* (2002). This book is full of beautiful photos of water crystals that can be enlarged for students to focus on as they listen to the meditation music supplied on the CDs. The photos are of water crystals that were made by exposing water in glasses while playing these pieces of music and then freezing them. The water crystal photographs in the book were taken after each piece of music contained in the CD was played to distilled water. The tip of the frozen and expanded ice produced a water crystal.

Dr Emoto believed in vibrational energy, and that as research progresses, it will be possible to heal the body with specific music compositions. I have used these photos and accompanying music with students, and it has helped them to focus. The photos of the crystals and the music allows for some focused meditation. It is also possible to use any piece of artwork or pictures of nature itself for students to focus on whilst listening to meditative music. If you are using YouTube for meditation music, they often have beautiful videos of nature to accompany the meditation.

Some teachers use colour instinctively when trying to create a mood for a piece of music. We all know that to be out in the green countryside relaxes us. It may be helpful to think of colour when you are trying to create an atmospheric background to the music you are playing for your students.

Cymatics and the cymascope for focused meditation

Cymatics is the study of sound waves and vibration of sound being made visible. Using cymatics, Swiss scientist Hans Jenny was able to show the effect of sound waves on solids and liquids. Jenny concluded that each individual cell generates its own sound; groups of cells also generate their own sounds, as do organs in the body. This body of evidence supports the influence of sound on health because cymatics proves that sound affects matter. Sir Peter Guy Manners collated the work that had been done in cymatics research and developed from it the therapy of cymatics. Dr Manners discovered how sound was instrumental in healing the body. He found that certain sound–tone combinations could help the functioning of each organ in the body. Each organ vibrates to its own frequency, which can be aided by the application of specific sound waves. Cymatics is used all over the world. There are now many different sound therapies that use this method.

John Stuart Reid realised that cymatics could assist his acoustic research and developed the cymascope, which allows sound to become visible in water when special lighting techniques are used. It produces a geometric pattern. Water appears to remember sonic frequencies imposed upon it. The cymascope app is now available in app stores for students to see sound come alive as visual patterns. A cymascope app is available from www.cymascope.com. This is particularly helpful to the profoundly deaf who will be able to see music. Cymascope patterns are accompanied by music or sounds and can be used with students for focused meditation. To see an example of cymascope in action, go to https://youtu.be/8uHZHol4ATA.

Tacpac and mindfulness

Some students enjoy the use of music and touch in a meditative way as with Tacpac. Tacpac is an activity that pairs music and touch to promote communication and social interaction, as well as sensory, neurological and emotional development. The music used is composed specifically to reflect the texture of each object so that the person receiving Tacpac experiences total sensory alignment. During Tacpac sessions, students are paired one on one with a familiar adult. Through linking familiar music consistently with objects, actions and people in a pattern of different activities, the partners communicate with each other. In Figure 5.3 you can see a student having a

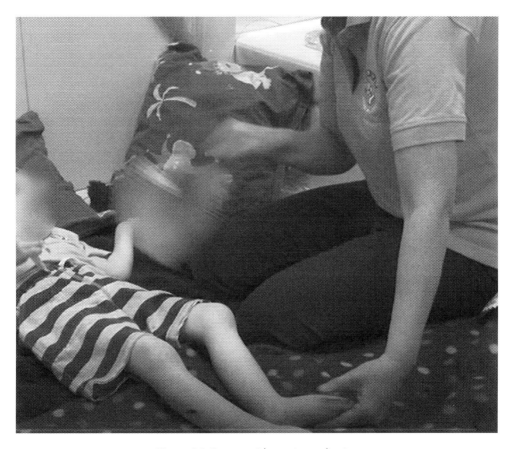

Figure 5.3 Tacpac with music meditation

pretty fan waved over him so that he feels its breeze as appropriate music accompanies the action. Tacpac provides a safe and structured framework for the 'receiving partner' to make contact with their own bodies, their environment and other people, and develop a relationship with these. The 'giving partner' ensures that each tactile experience is well organised and sensitively offered and adjusted to suit the receiving partner's responses.

For more information on Tacpac and the resources and training they provide, go to https://tacpac.co.uk/. Some special schools such as Three Ways special school in Bath make their own music selections and choose not to use the standard (commercially available) Tacpac music. If you visit YouTube, you can see a Tacpac session taking place at my previous school: https://youtu.be/7x4Tbgu2kcA?list=PL-a5MUplgl4nVMUEFGUGFg4jTxjvPyLur.

Sherborne therapy and mindfulness

I have also found that students with PMLD and SLD enjoy mindfulness that focuses on movement such as Sherborne therapy.

Staff and students from Ysgol Pen Coch helped produce a training DVD for the Sherborne Therapy Association. Sherborne is an approach to teaching and working with movement that

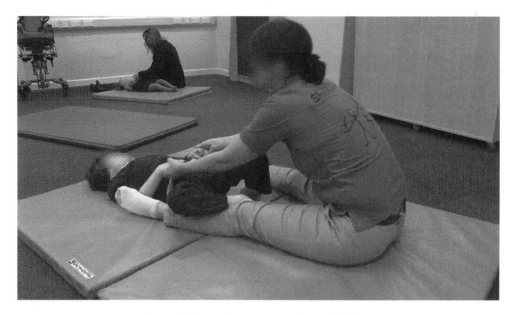

Figure 5.4 Sherborne with music meditation

is easily accessible to students with PMLD and SLD. It supports proprioception and mindfulness awareness of self and awareness of others. If you would like to be trained in Sherborne or want to find out more, go to www.sherbornemovementuk.org/about/sherborne-developmental-movement.

The approach is based on the philosophy and theory created by Rudolf Laban, the pioneer and founder of modern European dance and movement, and was devised by Veronica Sherborne after working closely with Laban for two years. Staff at different special schools that I have led or inspected have been trained to teach Sherborne dance therapy. Although the therapy is based on movement, we cannot underestimate the power that music has on the way that the student reacts. It has proved particularly useful for groups of students with SLD and ASD as well as groups of students with PMLD. If you visit YouTube, you can see a session taking place at my previous school that I had recorded: https://youtu.be/xqJ7Tmuscf8?list=PL-a5MUplgl4nVMUEFGUGF g4jTxjvPyLur.

Musico-kinetic therapy

This therapy uses both the trampoline and music. Research findings suggest that this therapy may be useful for improving the emotional condition of patients in a persistent vegetative state, especially those with severe brain damage (Anderson 2020b).

Let us now consider how music and vibrational sound contributes to sessions in the hydrotherapy pool.

6 Water and sound

Scientists believe that life on Earth began in the ocean, approximately four billion years ago. Water is a steady state between liquid and gas and covers over 70% of the earth. Sound is able to travel about four times faster and farther in water than it does in air. That is why whales can communicate over huge distances in the ocean. Sound cannot exist if it does not have something to travel through. Sound waves vibrate the molecules in matter. Water can be in a solid state of matter when it is frozen as ice and a gas state when it is heated as steam, and it is more often found in a liquid state. Sound vibrates in water. Music used in a pool of water has a different sound and effect to music used in a classroom.

We will see later in the chapter how the Halliwick approach uses songs as part of its therapy programme in the water; how liquid vibrations use vibrational sound through the water to stimulate the body; how Ai Chi uses music in its hydrotherapy sessions to develop rhythm in students; and how both body rhythm and music can be used in a hydrotherapy session through healing dance.

We will first look at what a hydrotherapy pool offers as a therapeutic intervention with music as a background stimulus.

Hydrotherapy

The hydrotherapy pool is used a great deal in special schools who are lucky enough to have them. The term hydrotherapy ('hydro' meaning water) refers to a process that uses water at any temperature or form to relieve pain and treat illness. This can mean having cold showers to improve health or alternatively having a warm bath to aid relaxation. A hydrotherapy pool is more about relaxation and so you should never find it cold. However, your pool manager should keep a close watch on the temperature to ensure it's at its optimum setting. Music has always been used during the delivery of hydrotherapy in every special school that I have worked in. I had this video taken to show how relaxing it is and how much the students enjoy it: https://youtu.be/czskF3O9Ix4?list=PL-a5MUplgI4nVMUEFGUGFg4jTxjvPyLur.

When I opened a new special school, Ysgol Pen Coch, in September 2009, three special schools had closed and all of the students (from age 2 to 11) from those schools were transferring

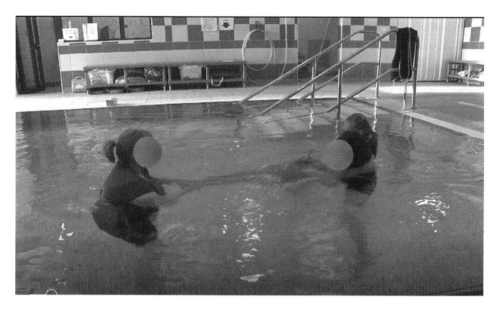

Figure 6.1 Hydrotherapy to music

to the new school. None of the schools had had a proper hydrotherapy pool and so it gave me the opportunity to start from scratch. I devised the policies and documents based on research and experience, having worked in three previous special schools that had hydrotherapy pools. I had also done a dissertation for my master's degree on the correct use of hydrotherapy pools. I ensured we had the right resources and that staff were trained in emergency procedures as well as in delivering hydrotherapy. A sound system in the pool area had been installed when the school was built which could deliver music while the students were in the pool or even while being changed for the pool, and different genres of music were bought so that we could find out which ones enhanced and stimulated each student's experience.

The students had never encountered hydrotherapy and we immediately had some positive results with some students suddenly being able to sleep through the night after experiencing a hydrotherapy session. Some of our students live with pain all of the time and their first time in the hydrotherapy pool may have been their first time without pain. Free from the restrictions of their wheelchair, leg braces or head support, they can manage often to move about independently and freely like they never can on land. To see the look of joy on their faces when they experience this for the first time is so rewarding. This physical and psychological well-being cannot be achieved anywhere else or in any other therapy. If you are having a new special school built, I highly recommend having a hydrotherapy pool installed.

The water is warmer than in an ordinary swimming pool, which helps to relax the muscles and reduce any muscle spasm. The heat of the water also enhances circulation of blood round the body, which is vital in speeding up the healing process. Mobility can be improved with hydrotherapy because people are able to perform activities in the pool that they are unable to perform on dry land. The support of the water and the reduced fear of falling onto a hard surface can aid mobility practice. Exercises against the resistance of water and dynamic exercises within the water can also improve muscle strength, balance and co-ordination.

Hydrotherapy can be used to speed up the recovery of students who are unable to weight-bear or can only partially weight-bear following surgery or injury, by increasing range of movement and maintaining muscle strength. Staff members and indeed county council members of staff have used our pool after having surgery to aid their recovery as well as students from all over the county. In addition to the above, hydrotherapy can:

- Increase mobility
- Reduce pain and muscle spasm
- Improve and maintain joint range of movement
- Strengthen weak muscle groups
- Increase physical fitness and functional tolerances
- Re-educate normal movement patterns
- Improve balance
- Improve co-ordination
- Improve posture
- Improve self-confidence
- Stimulate circulation
- Encourage communication
- Calm sensory needs

Hydrotherapy is an effective way to treat children with neurological and orthopaedic conditions. It is enjoyed by children with physical difficulties because it is fun and gives them a freedom of movement that can only be experienced in a hydrotherapy pool.

At all the special schools that I have worked in, programmes were devised by physiotherapists and followed by the hydrotherapy and support assistants.

Children who can weight-bear and do land-based physiotherapy programmes generally do not need to use a hydrotherapy pool. I have witnessed the misuse of a hydrotherapy pool where the water was reduced to swimming pool temperature and all students were encouraged to use it. This meant that often we could not get students with autism to leave the pool and students who would have benefited health-wise from the use of a heated hydrotherapy pool were fortunate if they got one session a week. In one instance, an assistant could not cope with the behaviours of a child with autism running around the pool and threw him in! Needless to say, she was dismissed, and police action was taken. You just need to prioritise the needs of your school. If you are going to use a hydrotherapy pool for students with sensory processing disorders, then you would need to ensure that you had a suitable policy to ensure it is being used correctly. Please see chapter 13 for a hydrotherapy policy you may adapt and copy. There would need to be a rigorous risk assessment drawn up and rules regarding entering and leaving the pool which would need to be strictly adhered to. Hydrotherapy is not swimming. A hydrotherapy pool is not a swimming pool. I have been reduced to tears when at one school the headteacher decided the pool was costing too much money, drained it, and stored old classroom furniture in it.

If you are lucky enough to have a hydrotherapy pool in your special school, I would ask you to do your research and use it for its intended purpose. At my last school, where I was headteacher, the pool was used across the authority by students with physical health needs in both mainstream and special schools. It was also used in the evenings by learning-disabled adults. They were only allowed to use the pool if we had a letter of support from a registered physiotherapist. The pool was in constant use throughout the week during the day and the evening. Our students with PMLD or with physical disabilities were able to use the pool as often as recommended by their physiotherapist. (Students with physical disabilities can have sensory processing disorders as well, by the way). That is how a hydrotherapy pool should be used. Students who do not have physical disabilities need to be prepared for real life and going to their local swimming pool by attending swimming sessions at the pool local to the school with supportive school staff. If, however, you do not have students with physical disabilities in your school but you do have students with sensory processing disorder, and you can afford a hydrotherapy pool for them, then obviously they are going to enjoy what it has to offer, particularly if you have one with multisensory applications. It is all about prioritising and creating the right documentation.

My hydrotherapy pool manager in North Wales (Emma) told me:

> For the past 6 years I have been working full time in the hydrotherapy pool, working with pupils and adults with a range of physical impairments. Many of the pupils/adults using the pool often have difficulty in controlling their movements and this can result in stiffness, floppiness,, unsteadiness, and unwanted involuntary movements. The warmth of the water enables the pupil/adult to do gentle stretching, floatation, and relaxing exercises – which are a lot more manageable when carried out in a heated pool. Music is always played as an additional relaxation technique. The children have specific musical preferences and we pander to them to ensure they have an enjoyable experience and do their exercises. Some pupils struggle to tolerate stretches and exercises for any length of time on dry land but will happily tolerate exercises in the water while relaxing or fun music is played.
>
> I have witnessed many physical benefits of the hydrotherapy pool, increased circulation, reduced muscle spasms, strengthened muscles and the relief of pain. Just seeing the pupil/ adult happy, relaxed, smiling and being free to move independently in the water is truly rewarding. For a pupil/adult to get out of their wheelchair and have the opportunity to change their body position and find freedom of movement and independence brings about physical and psychological well-being which cannot be achieved elsewhere. The ability for pupils/ adults to be independent in the water to achieve skills that may be difficult or impossible on land can only have favourable and lasting psychological effects which boost confidence and aid vocalisation. I have witnessed pupils/adults walking in the pool with extraordinarily little support from staff.
>
> Most of the pupil's IEP targets that we work on in the hydrotherapy pool are physical or communication targets, e.g. to reach out and touch an object (floating nearby), to communicate 'more' and to enjoy taking part in action rhymes and breathing techniques such as humming and blowing, with assistance. The advanced multisensory equipment that we have installed in the hydrotherapy pool, including lights, music, bubble machine, and the ICT switch, also enables pupils to reach targets, e.g. to use the switch to change the lights or to activate a piece of chosen music.

Music targets can be taken from the SOI framework and worked on during a session in the water.

Aquatic participation, at any level, can improve flexibility, endurance, cardiorespiratory function and strength, while helping reduce body fat – all components of being physically fit.

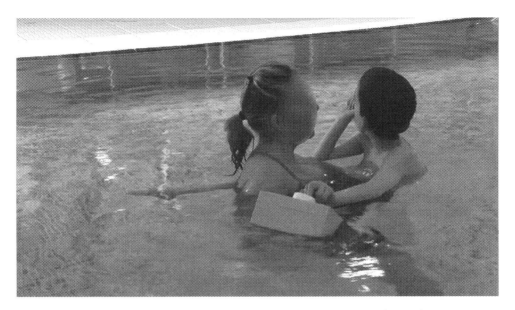

Figure 6.2 Activating a piece of chosen music safely from the pool

Halliwick approach

All of the staff I have worked with in special schools who use the hydrotherapy pool have been trained in the Halliwick approach. Songs and games are often used in the Halliwick approach and it is a fun time to be in the water. Halliwick games in the pool represent a great time to encourage oral skills, learn songs and encourage social interaction between staff and students. When our students suddenly have the freedom of movement that water gives them, they often find the ability to communicate more.

When I was deputy head of an 11–19 special school, my class of students, who all had PMLD, went in the hydrotherapy pool with my staff and me three times a week and we really enjoyed using Halliwick games and songs along with their physiotherapy programmes. When you go in the pool that much in a week, every week, you need to keep an eye on your costume. Wheeling a student back to class one day, with a towel thankfully around my lower half, I was told by a male member of staff in the corridor that my costume had become see through! When I became head of a special school, I made sure that my pool staff had costumes bought for them by the school on a regular basis. If at all possible, I would also recommend that you find time to change before leaving the changing area. To find out more about the Halliwick approach, go to www.halliwick. org.uk.

Liquid Vibrations

Liquid Vibrations is a charitable company that uses the different techniques that Emma describes but includes underwater music installation to enhance the well-being of students with disabilities.

The specialist speakers are installed to enable the music and sounds to be heard underwater. The company Liquid Vibrations provides:

* Training for schools who have hydrotherapy pools – staff and parents
* Help to implement practice into the curriculum
* Research and sharing of methodology
* Bespoke musical hydrotherapy sessions
* Taster sessions for teachers and families

To find out more, go to www.liquidvibrations.org.uk.

The quality of sound underwater is altered, in comparison to sound in the air, particularly through the vibrations that are caused within the water. Music vibrations are not only perceived by the ears but also the body. Check out 'Musical Hydrotherapy in practice – Bedelsford School' from Joel Cahen on Vimeo. The video is available at https://vimeo.com/334753698.

Ai Chi

Ai Chi is a form of aquatic exercise to music that has been adapted for students with PMLD and SLD. It is designed to strengthen and tone the body while also promoting relaxation and a healthy mind–body relationship. The technique was developed in Japan in 1993 by Jun Kunno, and it is practised all over the world.

Ai Ch is supposed to create a bond between the music, the movement and the adult partner. Limiting verbal language allows the child to focus on the rhythm and produce smoother motor responses. Gestural or gentle physical cues (tactile input) assist the child who may have limited body awareness.

The 16 foundation postures of Ai Chi can be transformed into an endless series of movements tailored to meet the needs of participants.

To see if Ai Chi could benefit your students and to look at research that supports it, visit www.clinicalaichi.org.

Healing dance

Healing dance is an aquatic technique involving music and movement developed by Alexander George in 1993. The website www.healingdance.org introduces you to the techniques and provides testimonials from teachers working with students who have special needs. You can buy MP4 healing dance instructional music videos and find out about training from the website.

Students learn to create the sensation of lightness and weightlessness, to generate a rhythmic field and to find the various 'rhythms of awareness'. Contact Alexander George for more information on where you can attend courses.

There is no doubt in my mind that music vibrates differently in a hydrotherapy pool full of water. Now we will look at how music vibrations can affect water inside the body.

Vibration and the feel of sound

Water makes up between 65% and 78% of our body (depending on age), comprising over 60% of our brain, heart, skin, muscles, kidneys, lungs and liver. For a developing foetus, surrounded by water, the intrauterine world is a world largely of sound. The eardrums and skin are believed to be the first sensory organs to develop in the foetus. The foetus lives daily with the mother's heart-beat and vibrating breathing. It is not surprising, therefore, that the vibrations of sound, as used in vibro-acoustic therapy, and passing through our bodies, affect our bodies. It is because they are mostly made up of water.

It may be useful, if we want students or even other members of staff to understand the effects of sound, vibration and music on the body, to demonstrate to those capable of understanding, a visual representation of these effects – as Chladni demonstrates.

Chladni resonance plates are metal plates that vibrate. Sand or salt is placed on the plate which is connected to a tone generator. The plate is attached to a speaker. When the music is played, depending on the vibrational frequency of the music, the sand particles move into different geometric patterns and, as the pitch of tone increases, the patterns become more complex. YouTube shows many Chladni experiments. To watch an experiment or show such an experiment to students, go to www.youtube.com/watch?v=1yaqUl. Ernest Chladni, who discovered this visual representation of vibrational sound, was an 18th century German physicist.

Vibro-acoustic therapy

The number of vibrations per second is known as the frequency. Frequency is measured in hertz (Hz); 1 Hz = 1 vibration per second. Vibro-acoustic therapy functions at 20 Hz to 100 Hz. The therapy uses sound to produce vibrations that are applied directly to the body. Since the human body is approximately 70% water and since sound travels five times more efficiently through water than through air, sound frequency stimulation is a highly efficient means for total body stimulation at a deep cellular level. Various tissue and muscles have their own vibration frequencies, which react in sympathetic resonance to sound stimuli. Specific vibrational frequencies can be used during the therapy. Through resonance phenomena, blood circulation and metabolic processes intensify, muscles release tension, and the body temperature increases. Anyone can experience and feel the vibrational benefits of sound.

Vibro-acoustic therapy provides massage therapy to muscles and joints that hand/mechanical massage cannot reach. For comparison purposes, ultrasound is a well-known and accepted sound technology for viewing tissue inside a body, and it operates at 20 kHz plus.

The development of vibro-acoustic therapy

We have known about and used vibro-acoustic therapy since 1980. The equipment used has continuously evolved since it was first developed by the Norwegian teacher, Olav Skille. He explored the use of vibro-acoustic stimulation for severely disabled children with whom he worked. It has mainly been used in the health service and through private practice, but there is no reason why it cannot be used in schools. I have found it particularly beneficial to students in a special school setting.

Below Olav Skille explains the basic idea of all vibro-acoustic therapy:

> We all know that the body is exposed to sound massage. It is so common that we seldom give this fact a thought. When we speak or sing, we produce sounds, and the vibrations from these sounds can be felt if we place our hands on the chest, back, larynx or the top of the skull of the person who is vocalising. These vibrations are not dangerous for the human being. It even may be so that these vibrations are of vital importance for us if we are to develop physically and mentally in a healthy way.
>
> The same kinds of vibrations are transferred to the body during vibro-acoustic therapy. The only difference is that the source of sound is external, and that the sound sources are spread over a larger physical area. Thus, all parts of the body can receive the same amount of vibrations simultaneously.
>
> (Skille 2013)

In order for the body to receive and be able to understand and respond to the vibrations, specific frequencies are used to obtain a specific effect. This is pure vibro-acoustic therapy, or VAT. For example, according to the research done by Olav Skille (more than 40 years of research), we know that low frequencies from 40 Hz to 86 Hz can be used with success to treat conditions ranging from circulatory problems to asthma. He has produced many papers providing evidence of improvement in students with PMLD, autism, constipation, insomnia and physical difficulties with professional contributions from around the world (Skille 2007). Research by Dr Suzanne Jonas of the USA has shown that frequencies as low as 30 Hz have a tremendously positive impact on patients with Parkinson's disease (Jonas 2011).

I was headteacher of Ysgol Pen Coch in North Wales from 2009 to 2019. In 2014 I set up a vibro-acoustic therapy room that contained a waterbed (donated by a local charity) that was then embedded with speakers or transducers which transmit sinusoidal sound waves bathing the student repeatedly through vibrations. In 2017, due to the popularity of the therapy, we added to this and purchased vibro-acoustic systems that could also be used independently in classrooms.

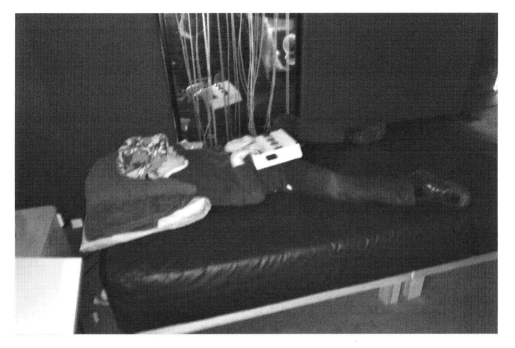

Figure 7.1 Vibro-acoustic waterbed in use
Student activating coloured lights whist receiving vibro-acoustic therapy.

Contraindications

Vibro-acoustic therapy is very safe therapy because it is based on low frequency sound vibration which we are all affected by in our ordinary everyday life. However, there are certain conditions we need to be mindful of, and a screening form (please find a photocopiable form in the Resources chapter) must be completed by parents and consent given by a doctor before a student can start VAT.

Resources

We used specially developed and patented Somatron CDs available from Somatron.com. The Somatron Corporation was founded in 1985 by Byron Eakin in the USA. We bought all of the CDs and these were played through the waterbed. Somatron's CD system is designed for settings and procedures that require deep relaxation, pain relief and stress reduction. Somatron (see Section 19 of the Appendix) claim that Dr George Patrick, who conducted an NIH study, reported a 53% aggregate reduction in a variety of symptoms among 272 patients after each had experienced a 25-minute vibro-acoustic session using the composition 'Balance' (CD Level 1).

You can use these CDs to reduce a person's level of stress and relieve their pain. We tried them out beforehand to familiarise ourselves with their therapeutic differences. The therapist fell asleep!

The CDs come with an instruction manual on how to design a programme, with step-by-step instructions as well as assessment forms, and evaluation support. I recommend looking at all of the CDs that Somatron offer. Therapists may contact other companies to get specially made vibrational sounds for specified conditions, e.g. VibLab software, made by a Finnish company that produces 25 premade treatment sound patterns. These can be stored on your computer. The sound is transferred to the computer audio output cable or wirelessly via a Bluetooth connection. Using VibLab software you can give treatments, for example with Multivib, Nextwave and Taikofon products. To find out more, contact Pekka@viblab.fi.

If VAT therapy CDs are used for ordinary auditive listening, the listener may feel nausea, dizziness and psychophysical uneasiness if the listening goes on for some time. These programmes are made for use in vibro-acoustic chairs/beds only in order to transfer therapeutic sound vibrations directly to the human body. The programmes are *not* intended for listening purposes.

Please see chapter 12 for a vibro-acoustic policy you may wish to adapt and copy.

Alternative VAT methods

The vibro-acoustic therapy system (music in-built) available from www.soundoasis.com/products/sleep-sound-therapy-systems/vibroacoustic-therapy-system/ is a shaped back cushion that can be used on its own with small students or nested into a chair surround for larger students to relax into. This vibro-acoustic therapy system was developed by Dr Lee Bartel who gives a TED Talk on the benefits of the system. Visit https://youtu.be/wDZgzsQh0Dw to find out more. We had two of these in addition to the waterbed.

Multivib, a Norwegian company, also sell vibro-acoustic equipment. To find out more, go to www.multivib.com/multivib-products/.

Flexound, a Finnish company, provide augmented audio equipment. To find out more, go to https://flexound.com/. Taikofon is a product of Flexound Systems (www.taikofon.com/).

Another Finnish company use the name physioacoustic instead of vibro-acoustic, but the principles are the same – though they are at the top end of the price market. They can be contacted for more information at info@nextwaveworldwide.com.

Training

Basic training can be provided by Soundbeam trainers. Members of staff and I were trained by the Soundbeam staff and this just takes an hour or so. They provided us with a booklet to use. If you choose to use Soundbeam, they will leave you with a booklet.

I also paid privately so that I could be trained by VIBRAC. VIBRAC is the Skille–Lehikoinen Centre for Vibroacoustic Therapy and research based in Finland. VIBRAC training is more intensive training. It is the only body worldwide offering certified evidence-based further education courses in vibro-acoustic therapy.

The first level of training lasts two days with 14 hours of contact sessions and 14 hours of independent work. This underpins any practical work you intend to do during the second level.

The second level is made up of three modules. Module 1 lasts four days and consists of lectures, demonstrations, exercises and discussions. Module 2 lasts three months and it is client/student-based work which forms your studies and reports. Module 3 lasts four days and is supervised. If you pass you become a registered practitioner with VIBRAC.

There is a gap between doing levels 2 and 3 while you consolidate your practice and you may decide not to go on to level 3. However, it may be cost-effective as a school to train a member of staff to level 3 and then recoup money spent on training and travel costs by training staff in other schools.

The third level is the advanced level and you must have clinical practice and experience to take this training. It lasts four days. It consists of lectures, demonstrations, exercises, discussions and case consultation. You can opt to become a VAT trainer and supervisor for VIBRAC once you attain this level.

It does depend on financing as to which levels you can afford to do. Level 1 is sufficient to deliver the therapy in a school. If you wish to have your own practice, then the other levels are beneficial. In recent months level 1 has become web-based so there is no need to travel to Europe and find somewhere to board. Levels 2 and 3 at this present time require attendance at a venue in Europe, and these venues and dates are advertised on the VIBRAC website regularly: https://www.vibrac.fi/.

Assessment

Vibro-acoustic therapy treatment itself should be based on an assessment. Goals can then be set for the treatment and a plan developed in line with the student's health needs and IEP. The plan has to be monitored and evaluated throughout the therapy process (including possible consultation with the multi-disciplinary team). An example of an assessment is a visual analogue scale (see chapter 13 for a copy you can use).

Why have you decided a student requires the therapy? Is it to improve their quality of life? Is it to help them manage their anxieties and stress levels? Is it to alleviate pain? Is it to support their sleep patterns and aid insomnia? There should be a pre-therapy discussion with the parent (and if appropriate the student), and a post-therapy discussion or completion of evaluation form (see chapter 13) to ensure the student is benefiting and to monitor its effectiveness in reaching the goals set. Therapeutic interventions should have an outcome. Yes, they can be a pleasurable experience, but any inspection team will say, 'So what?' You will need to show that it has made a difference to the students' quality of life and that hopefully it will have impacted on their ability to learn.

Listening to additional music

How do you choose music for students to listen to while having vibro-acoustic therapy? It must be remembered that the vibrational music used during the therapy is not meant to be heard. The volume on the vibro-acoustic output should not be too high, as the sound therapy is not based on volume but on frequency. If it is decided that a student will benefit from additional music to listen to, then you must have a clear idea of the function of the music. What kind of music do you want to use?

There are four categories of music to choose from:

* Relaxing music which has a slow, calm, soothing tempo with predictable, safe, soft tones and timbre
* Imagery evoking music which activates images and triggers pleasant emotion
* Entertaining music which is neutral, not moving or stimulating but more than just silence
* Disturbing music, which is irritating and evokes annoying images, not suitable for this therapy

You should aim to get to know the student's likes and dislikes, as use of preferred music can be useful and can create a feeling of familiarity and safety at the beginning of the therapy process. Students have quite diverse tastes; sometimes adolescents prefer fast tempo and it actually relaxes them. I have found that in 90% of cases the students preferred silence and enjoyed feeling the vibrational frequencies. Many of them fell asleep. It can even play its part in focused meditation. When I extended the use of the school for the evenings for adults with learning disabilities, carers brought in relaxing music for the adults to listen to while they received the therapy. It was a popular therapy with the adults, with one adult choosing the therapy three times a week, as he was able to sleep afterwards.

Delivery

The therapy can be completely controlled by the therapist according to the assessment needs and the therapy can be delivered in conjunction with the student input (if they are able to communicate). The therapy can be followed up at home and delivered by an adult who has been trained in its use if the home is able to purchase the equipment needed. In a private practice ten sessions might be offered. In a school it depends on the continuous assessment of need and the waiting list of students.

Vibro-acoustic therapy should always be applied in a systematic manner. The therapy assistant or practitioner providing the therapy ensures that the student feels secure and is prepared for the session and that the CD is not turned on until the student is comfortable on the bed and the environment aids relaxation. A pillow is positioned behind the student's head for comfort. A blanket is provided, as the treatment can involve the loss of body heat. The treatment lasts between 20 and 30 minutes. It is not unusual for the student to fall asleep during the session. It may take a little while for a student to adjust after such a deeply relaxing form of therapy.

A session sheet/evaluation form (see chapter 13) is completed in an unobtrusive manner and the targets for the session relate either to an IEP assessment target or a well-being target agreed with the class teacher. The assistant is incredibly careful with her choice of words and tone of voice and endeavours to build a trusting, sensitive, therapeutic relationship. The evaluation forms completed by parents and/or teachers already suggest that students are better able to participate when they return to their classes.

The vibro-acoustic sounds are not heard by the student but felt. Various tissue and muscles have their own vibration frequencies, which react in sympathetic resonance to sound stimuli.

We have used the therapy with students and adults with learning disabilities who have autism, ADHD, cerebral palsy, aphasia, asthma, anxiety, insomnia, emotional and behavioural difficulties (EBD), undergoing cancer treatment or recovering from surgery. The benefits gained are reported to include the relief of muscle tension, an increase in body awareness, the stimulation of circulation, the diminishing of constipation problems, reductions in anxiety and success in screening out sounds that may otherwise be upsetting to some students.

It is not suitable for those suffering with low blood pressure or anti-inflammatory conditions, and a screening form should be completed before a session is allowed to proceed (see chapter 13).

It can be used as a multi-modal approach, whereby the therapist works with the student or adult on physiological and psychological experiences, taking the mind–body approach – though the person would need to be of sufficient cognitive ability and able to communicate.

Often, we think of stress as something which affects us only in a mental capacity but in addition to these psychological problems it can also cause a multitude of physical issues. We already know that stress-related illnesses can cause high blood pressure, headaches, insomnia, depression, etc. which all have a knock-on effect on the immune system. We trained a therapist to deliver vibro-acoustics in the evenings at our school. She noticed that adults suffering stress, anxiety and depression open up more and communicated more freely when using vibro-acoustic therapy. She also used the recommended Somatron CDs which deal with many different themes. She was so taken by the results of vibro-acoustic therapy at our school that she gave up her job and opened up her own vibro-acoustic practice locally.

Vibro-acoustic therapy is most often used in hospitals and private practice, but more schools have taken it on board and I know that since I have given talks at educational conferences about its benefits other special schools have introduced it into their schools. Some of the benefits we have found:

* Students learn to relax
* Staff have used it to relax after work
* It has helped with pain relief; we have even had a young child with terminal cancer from mainstream school tell us of its benefits to him
* Spasticity reduction
* Alleviating neurological symptoms
* Relieving stress symptoms
* Developing body awareness
* Relieving constipation
* Supporting creative processing
* It is a holistic approach

Benefits

For years it has been recognised that relaxation accelerates healing and enhances the immune system, but as the public has grown cautious about the side effects of pharmaceuticals, the medical community is turning increasingly to music as a non-drug stress reduction strategy.

The psychiatric drugs industry makes millions of pounds every year. Drugs do not change fundamental brain activity and work only as long as the patient keeps taking them.

Students in special schools are sometimes given drugs such as Ritalin which can make them drowsy and unable to actively take part in learning. I passionately believe that as special educators it is our job to ensure that our students are in the best frame of mind to learn. That is not possible with such drugs.

As I write I am reminded of a ten-year-old boy with severe autism we had in a school where I was headteacher. He had, over the years that he attended our school, tuned in to the therapeutic and technological interventions that he found benefit from. When he could feel a red mist descend, he would either come looking for me and take my hand to guide us to the vibro-acoustic therapy room, or take himself there. His parents told me that if he had not had the opportunity to experience the different therapies on offer and have the use of the latest technology, he was on his way to being prescribed Ritalin.

If we can deliver therapeutic interventions from an early age to students in special schools, they might not need to deaden their senses with drugs.

I had a session filmed if you wish to see vibro-acoustic therapy in practice supporting a student with PMLD: https://youtu.be/Ocp1buvwSS8?list=PL-a5MUplgI4nVMUEFGUGFg4jTxjvPyLur.

We have seen how the frequency of sound can have a positive effect on health and well-being and we will continue to look at positive effects – but also some of the negative effects – of the frequencies of sound in the next chapter.

8 Health, well-being and sound

Vibrational sound

To understand why vibrational sound is now used in some special schools for health and well-being, we need to understand what vibrational sound is.

Albert Einstein (n.d.) predicted that 'future medicine will be the medicine of vibration'. Einstein himself was a classical violinist, having studied the violin from the age of five. In his later years he was vice president of Princeton University's symphony orchestra between 1952 and 1955. In one of his late journals he wrote, 'If I were not a physicist, I would probably be a musician. I often think in music. I see my life in terms of music. I get most joy in life out of music.'

Using vibrations and sound for health and well-being has existed for many years, as this chapter will show. Advances in technology and Einstein's $E=MC^2$ gave us a new way of looking at health and well-being, based on vibration and energy. Today, considering quantum physics, our understanding reflects the paradigm of our time. Society is not as dismissive as it was in the time of Royal Rife (see Section 16 of the Appendix) for example.

Sound is vibration caused by something or someone which travels through the medium of a gas, a liquid or a solid. It cannot move through the environment without those carrier objects. As a rule, when we hear something, we are sensing the vibrations it makes in the air. The eardrum then vibrates when the vibrations reach it. The brain converts these vibrations into sound. Everything resonates. Even a table has a vibrational frequency. Sometimes we can hear a frequency, sometimes we cannot.

String theory suggests that everything in the universe is made up of vibrating strings of energy. Just as the strings on a violin have resonant vibrations at which they prefer to vibrate – the same is true for string theory (Greene 2000). Particle properties in string theory are the musical patterns of fundamental loops of string. One vibrational sound can tune the other, train it into harmony, as in entrainment.

The concept of vibrational musical harmonies in the universe, intrinsically alive within the spacing of the planets, existed in medieval philosophy and was often called the 'music of the spheres'. In his book *Harmonices Mundi* (published in 1619), Johannes Kepler discusses the physical harmonies in planetary motion. In his book he represented the planets as musical tones. 'And who has been made drowsy by the very sweet harmony of the planets begins to dream.' (Kepler 1997)

If we think of the universe as vibrational energy, then what of Planet Earth, and how do vibrational energy and sound frequencies affect us? It is more than plausible that humans and various Earth life forms are tuned or resonate to the Schumann vibrations of the Earth-ionosphere cavity (see Section 11 of the Appendix). Research in Russia has also confirmed this phenomenon (Vladimirsky et al. 1995). This technological age poses questions as to technology's effect on the Schumann vibrations and ultimately the effect that technological interference with those musical harmonies of the universe have on our health and well-being (Anderson 2020a). Meklit Hadero, a singer-songwriter, said in her TED Talk, 'A healthy environment has animals and insects taking up low, medium and high frequency bands in exactly the same way as the symphony (orchestra) does'.

She also said, 'The world is alive with musical expression. We are already immersed.' (www.youtube.com/Watch?v=NAkkckxE9i8)

In his TED Talk Julian Treasure says:

> Music is not the only sound that can affect your emotions. Natural sound can do that too. Birdsong, for example, is a sound that most people find reassuring. There's a reason for that: over hundreds of thousands of years we've learned that when the birds are singing, things are safe.
>
> (www.youtube.com/Watch?V=rRepnhXq33s)

Positive effects of sound and vibration on health and well-being

The technological age that we find ourselves in and the exponential rate of emerging technologies using sound and vibration, such as focused ultrasound and the use of certain algorithms, allow for innovative medical procedures unavailable and unthinkable a hundred years ago. Has man managed to harness sound frequency purely for the good of mankind?

Those of us who have been fortunate enough to have had children since the 1980s have had ultrasound scans that show us images of the developing foetus. These images come from bouncing ultrasonic sound waves at the desired area using a transducer probe and detecting the echoes that bounce back. Humans are not able to hear the sound as it is above our audible range of hearing.

Ultrasound in now also routinely used in medicine to heal certain conditions and specific complaints. John Grisham, best-selling author of legal thrillers such as *The Pelican Brief*, has written an easy-to-read book about the use of focused ultrasound (Grisham 2016). It is a free e-book called *The Tumour* and Grisham believes it is the most important book that he has ever written. Grisham has been a board member of the Focused Ultrasound Foundation for years.

High intensity focused ultrasound (HIFU) is now used to destroy tumours but cannot be currently used to treat widespread cancers.

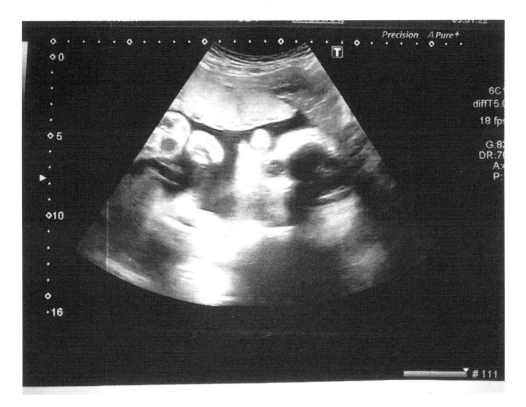

Figure 8.1 Ultrasound scan, Morgan Chaplin, 18 January 2016

Sound frequency healing

In his TED Talk, Dr Anthony Holland, a renowned music-composer-turned-cancer-researcher, describes how an opera singer can shatter glass by hitting just the right high-pitched note. He goes on to explain how his research targeted cancer cells in the same way with an electronic frequency machine. This is not new and in 1934 Royal Raymond Rife was able to cure 16 people of terminal cancer using his sound frequency machine. The resonant frequencies, known as oscillating, pulsed electric field (OPEF), lead to changes in the shape of the cells and eventual destruction (as described by Dr Holland in his TED Talk, linked below). A specifically tuned sound wave vibrates the nucleolus membrane of a cancer cell to the point of rupture. The method should leave healthy cells unharmed while non-invasively destroying the diseased cancer cells. Dr Holland gives a TED Talk on shattering cancer with resonant frequencies music: www.youtube.com/watch?v=1w0_kazbb_U.

Dr Holland says in his TED Talk that he hopes that these vibratory frequencies will one day be the norm for cancer care.

The use of sound frequency for health and well-being is not new. Scientists, researchers, musicians and the like today can reflect on the significant work of people like Huygens, Tesla, Abrams, Lakhovsky, Rife and Oster. (See the Appendix for more information.) Those pioneers have thankfully left some of their work behind so that during this time of enlightenment, when our understanding reflects the paradigm of our time, we have the technology to further develop the use of vibration and sound in the field of health and well-being further. Students in schools get to learn about and experience the effects of vibration and sound upon the world and the individual. We need to tread carefully. We now know that everything we do every day has an impact on the planet.

Research and historical evidence show us that sound, vibration and music can indeed have an effect upon the organs of the body. Chapters in this book introduce the reader to different therapies, technologies and specific frequencies that have been shown to have a positive effect for some students on their health and well-being and sometimes on their learning. Yet we are all different. No two people are exactly alike and what works for one person may not work for someone else.

Hypersensitivity to sound

When a musician plays a note of a certain pitch, the musical instrument vibrates. The number of vibrations per second is known as the frequency. Once again, frequency is measured in hertz (Hz); 1 Hz = 1 vibration per second. A piece of music produces a complex pattern of sound waves made up of many different frequencies. Frequencies of sound have been proven to influence people's mental health.

Some frequencies can tune the brain better for learning whilst some low and even high frequency sounds can upset and have an unhealthy effect. This is because the human ears are capable of hearing sounds with frequencies as low as 20 Hz and as high as 20,000 Hz (20 kHz). However, this range decreases with age (Leventhall 2009).

We are living in a constant unseen smog of man-made devices emitting low-level frequency sounds, and those hypersensitive to sound frequency could be affected by any or all of these frequencies. Electro-sensitivity is now recognised by the World Health Organization (WHO 2005) but the only country in the world acknowledging and helping its sufferers is Sweden (Hallberg et al. 2006).

Sound at frequencies below 20 Hz is called infrasound; these are ultra-low frequencies that we cannot hear but can be felt as vibration. However, some people can be affected by this ultra-low frequency which can appear as stress of unknown cause. Low frequency sounds are low-pitched hums or drones and can be the central heating system, fridges, machinery, etc. It can even come from the sea. High frequency, including high-pitched noises such as ringing and whistling, may also be troublesome for some people.

Sometimes sounds become scary because we are not expecting them – a knock on the door late at night, an ambulance siren on the street outside. Everyone experiences problems with sounds they find unpleasant: maybe it is the scrape of chalk on a blackboard, the pneumatic drill in the road works outside our home or maybe a baby crying on a crowded train or bus. That is quite normal. What is not normal is when this becomes a daily or hourly occurrence, and when it starts to interfere with your life.

Auditory hypersensitivity, or hypersensitivity to sound, may include sensitivity to specific triggering noises, or loud noises in general. Babies who are hypersensitive to sound might cry constantly because of this sensitivity. Students with auditory hypersensitivity can experience distress upon hearing the triggering sound. Sometimes the complaint can be traced to a sound source, but for those of us not tuned into that low frequency wave it can be difficult to ascertain the problem. Low frequencies have a stronger oscillatory wave to the brain through the skull and other bones. We know that there are many natural phenomena, some animals, and machines such as air conditioners that produce low frequency sounds (Cody 1996).

Students with autism are often in the fight, flight or freeze mode. If a student suffers from a sensory processing difficulty linked to hearing, then they could be tuned into a low or high frequency sound and get into a fight, flight or freeze mode when they hear that sound, which signals a perceived threat to their survival.

This can be distressing, because to the sufferer the sound could appear to be loud, even deafening, whereas others cannot hear it. If they begin to associate a sound with a threat, then this 'alerting' reaction takes place. It could be that this survival mechanism is triggered in sufferers (whether or not they are conscious of it), and places them in a constant state of alert so that they may not even be able to sleep.

For some students it is a regular noise that we hear every day which ordinary people are able to tune out, but which they are unable to – perhaps on a par with someone suffering from tinnitus. If there are any health effects, it would appear that they are the result of the reaction to the sound rather than the sound itself. This is because the sound does not appear to affect the majority of people. However, the stress felt is real. Cortisone and adrenaline pump through the body causing unpleasant physical tension. It can cause a life of isolation, as the student wishes to avoid the noises that cause this effect on their body.

Supporting students who are sound sensitive

If the noise itself cannot be controlled, then the best option for the parent, student or class teacher is to try to control their reaction to the noise. Some ways are:

- Recognise the triggers, if possible. Each time your child/student becomes agitated due to noise, note it down – what was the cause, how did he behave, what, if anything, helped?
- Prepare your child/student in advance if you know you are going to encounter a sound they cannot tolerate. Sometimes just knowing can be enough.
- Distract (you may find a student will try their own distraction techniques such as stimming – see Section 18 of the Appendix) with enjoyable activities/calming techniques/fidgets.
- Use ear defenders or ear plugs.
- Use meditation downloads or apps.
- Use earphones to listen to a favourite music or a book.
- Set up quiet zones in school so that the student may go to them when overwhelmed.

- Use white noise (free apps are available – try https://www.techjunkie.com/best-free-white-noise-apps-android).
- At some cinemas and theatres, the front desk will supply you with headphones to listen to the event, ensuring the student can only hear what they have chosen to hear.
- Find a therapeutic intervention that your child/student enjoys and use it.
- Get enough sleep. Melatonin, a hormone made in the brain, is a powerful antioxidant that secretes at night while you sleep. This hormone is vital in repairing the body. Some students with autism/ADHD and other learning difficulties whom I have worked with over the years have been prescribed melatonin. There is a useful article on its benefits that I recommend – Rossignol and Frye (2011).
- On the other hand, some students with a sensory processing disorder are hyposensitive to sound. They may prefer to be in loud settings and try to create noise whenever possible. They might slam doors, play with loud toys and make noises any way that they can. This requires careful management, as their desire for sound can impact on other students' need for quiet. Some ways of assisting them to have noise stimulation are:

  - Earphones are a great help, if they will tolerate wearing them, as they can listen to their favourite noises and tunes without disturbing others.
  - A music room where the student can go and play drums or other instruments can help.
  - Find a therapeutic intervention that your child/student benefits from and use it.

There are many different therapies and interventions explored in this book that can help the student.

Hearing loss

Make provision for those who cannot hear sound, for the deaf and hearing impaired in schools – include regular visits by a Speech and Language Therapist, audiologists, a deaf signing instructor and a tutor. The continued merging of electronic innovation and hearing aid technology mean hearing aids become smaller, sleeker and smarter.

Different degrees and types of hearing loss, as well as differences in a student's ability to use the technology, will have an impact on the results, but technological progress has allowed users many practical benefits, such as wireless connectivity via Bluetooth. These assistive hearing devices are particularly helpful for people with hearing aids or cochlear implants to use in a T or loop setting. They can also be used by anyone with headphones or earphones. The use of this technology allows sound to be amplified so that the distinction of different pitches may be heard and developed. In this book I have mentioned the frequencies of sound and it is worth considering that those with hearing impairments may be able to hear certain frequencies.

Today audio quality listening environment and sound field systems are often installed in the classrooms where the hearing-impaired students work as well as a school hall. In my previous school we had all of this and I believe they should be installed in all schools. Any system that operates sound has to be well maintained in order for that sound to be heard clearly with no distortions.

In the introduction to this book I mention how Dame Evelyn Glennie feels sound and vibrations. Most deaf people become reliant on their other senses as a result of their hearing loss.

Rhythm, an important aspect of music, can be felt. Sometimes we need to forget the traditional ways of teaching music. As Ignacio Estrada is quoted as saying, 'If a child cannot learn the way we teach, then maybe we should teach the way they learn'. Maybe we need to teach music from a rhythm base to children who have hearing impairments. As teachers it is our duty to teach. In this day and age of enlightenment there can be no excuse for blaming a child for not being able to learn when it may well be our teaching style that is at fault.

There are ways of using sound and music to enhance learning and we will look at some of those in the next chapter.

The use of sound support in schools

Have you noticed the student who puts their hands over their ears or cries in response to loud sounds? Have you picked up on the student who seems to be daydreaming or lacking attention because they have tuned out of environmental noises; or, conversely, are so distracted by environmental sounds that they cannot concentrate? Have you noticed the student who learns better visually because they cannot cope with auditory instruction? Do you know a student who has a history of ear infections, is non-verbal or diagnosed language difficulties? Have you noticed the student who seems easily distracted but may in fact be hearing the overhead light fittings that you cannot hear? Finally, have you noticed the student who hums to himself to try to block out the noises he can hear.

We are constantly being influenced by sound, be it the song of a bird, the seashore, or a noisy classroom. Students with an auditory sensitivity may be hypersensitive to sound and be oversensitive to noises. One way of dealing with an oversensitivity to sound is to allow students to wear ear defenders. A high percentage of students at my previous schools used ear defenders when they needed to. Some schools also ensure that teaching and learning areas are carpeted to reduce reverberation of sound. It is also important to ensure that any technology being used is regularly maintained so that any sound produced has clarity.

Filtered Sound Training (FST), Auditory Integration Training (AIT) and sound therapy

AIT and FST have been used with students who have these issues. I believe it is something that can be delivered in schools today.

AIT and FST are educational music programmes aimed at helping students to listen more clearly and improve their learning ability. When there is no medical reason to explain their auditory sensitivity, it could be that the brain is not processing sounds well enough and this is where these programmes can help.

Auditory stimulation

On a weekend in 2015 I attended a tribute conference in London dedicated to Dr Guy Bérard. Bérard (1916–2014) was an accomplished ear, nose and throat (ENT) specialist and pioneer of the AIT intervention. He developed an approach begun by Dr Alfred Tomatis (1920–2001). Tomatis's research showed that the bones of the ear are the first to form in utero. The unborn child begins to hear its mother's voice from four and a half months. The Tomatis method of auditory stimulation was developed in the 1970s using music that has been electronically modulated and usually includes listening to a recording of the mother's voice.

Bérard believed that some individuals were hypersensitive to some frequencies compared to other frequencies, and so sounds that they heard could be magnified or distorted. This could cause them behavioural and cognitive problems. He developed AIT with the goal of removing this hypersensitivity so that the person can hear normally.

At the conference I listened to practitioners from all over the world, but the person whose speech affected me the most was Georgiana Stehli. Georgiana was diagnosed with autism from birth by reputable autism specialists in New York. She had the usual severe behavioural difficulties associated with autism because of her extreme hypersensitivity to certain sounds and situations. The family came upon AIT. This simple intervention was the turning point for Georgiana's emergence from autism and today she is a successful businesswoman and mother. Her mother wrote a book about the journey – *The Sound of a Miracle* (Stehli 1995).

At the conference Georgiana told us how on the way to school she could hear the drains of the local hotels and would cause a scene all the way to school. She could not communicate at the time and so could not let her parents know that she wasn't getting in a state because she didn't want to go to school but that she didn't want to go that way to school. If her parents took her to the seaside, she would have a meltdown. The waves made thunderous noises to her. In the classroom she could hear the noises the radiators made. Once she had AIT, she started to improve.

I am always looking for the key to enhance learning for those with a learning disability or difference. The same key does not work for every person with a learning difficulty because every person is different, with different DNA. If Geogiana was able to live a happier life because of AIT, then I wanted to see if AIT was a key some of my students could use. Hypersensitivity to sound is something that many students in special schools suffer with.

Introducing FST into the school

In 2015 I funded myself and trained in FST during my Easter break from school. It was a week-long intensive programme and I was extremely fortunate that Rosalie Seymour agreed to fly over from Qatar where she was working and train me in my own home. Rosalie Seymour was the first AIT trainer and practitioner in South Africa. She introduced FST, allowing effective AIT to be done in the home.

In April, our school purchased the FST equipment and I trained staff on how to deliver the training. FST is a method that uses music to re-train listening skills by filtering the sound in a specialised way. The student listens to pieces of music that essentially have random sounds missing which presents the brain with unpredictable sounds to process. It exercises the auditory system. It seems that in these training programmes the mechanisms of the ear receive a 'passive massage', and this has the effect of 'toning up' or 'tuning in' the listening mechanism. FST is offered in a personalised package of 20 half-hour sessions. These sessions are done twice a day consecutively for ten days. Changes that occur in listening and learning are seen over the period of four months following FST.

Assessing the effectiveness of FST

At our school we used the POPAT approach to phonics and the remediation of phonological disorders which teaches an in-depth understanding of speech sounds and their order in words before letters are introduced. It is used widely as a remedial programme for various speech and language difficulties in many special schools.

In April 2015 we found that a number of students had not made any progress with POPAT since September 2014, so we offered the parents of those students the opportunity for their child to undertake FST. We wanted to see whether FST would improve their listening ability. Hearing problems can affect behaviour, sensitivity to noises in the classroom, interaction with other students, and speech and language development. We wanted to have a way of measuring the learning progress of students using FST.

We decided to invite parents to find out more about the auditory training for themselves and gave them an introduction and online links to follow. If they wanted to go privately to have this training it would cost them upwards of £1,000. We were offering it for free, but they had to consult with their child's doctor and commit to delivering and picking their child up from school on the days that they receiveded the training.

Please see chapter 13 for the POPAT progress report. It is an incredibly positive report.

As well as the progress report, we had feedback from parents. All feedback was positive. Children were more aware and responsive and improved communication and language.

Several peer-reviewed journals for speech therapists and journals for autism have published studies into the validity of AIT. (For a critique of these studies, see www.georgianainstitute.org.)

If you wish to use music in your school in this way and wish to find out more, go to https://www.aitinstitute.org/ait_and_brain.htm, https://www.filteredsoundtraining.net/what-is-filtered-sound-training-fst/ or https://www.auditoryintegrationtraining.co.uk.

Sound therapy

Sound therapy is a therapy that supports auditory processing. Similar to AIT and FST, it enhances auditory processing. It is a listening programme for the ears and the brain. A passive programme of specially recorded sounds activates muscles in the middle ear, restoring function to this delicate mechanism and stimulating the auditory pathways to the brain. This helps improve natural coordination, learning and listening abilities. It can be used at home and there is a free e-book available for anyone to use. Go to https://youtu.be/5KNhesNod0I.

Here is a link to a video about the effects sound therapy had on a child with autism: https://youtu.be/4kUIv29MbvQ.

Some schools are nervous about using sound therapies as there is not a lot of published research to back up its effectiveness. I would suggest that you do your own research, as I did. Parents look for anything to help their child and will often pay a huge amount; but I believe it should be provided for free by an innovative and forward-thinking school. All care and risk assessments should be followed as with introducing any new therapy into a school.

The listening project

The listening project (Porges et al. 2014) was designed to reduce auditory sensitivities through exercising the neural regulations of the middle ear muscles. Filtered music was specifically designed and trials were conducted. Data from both trials confirmed that filtered music selectively reduced auditory hypersensitivities. The listening project has developed a middle ear sound absorption system (MESAS) to measure the middle ear transfer function. This will provide data to validate the effectiveness of the use of filtered sound. The Safe and Sound Protocol (SSP) is a five-hour auditory intervention programme based on the listening project; more information can be found at https://www.integratedlistening.com.

Soundwaves and neurofeedback

Through some of the therapies that we used at Ysgol Pen Coch children's behaviour was shown to improve. However, once their behavioural problems were under control their learning disabilities sometimes became more obvious. Even though therapies can help students to relax and be more ready to take part in education, their learning skills often need specialised help.

The brain tends to match its own soundwave pulses to those of exterior sound pulses in the environment, a phenomenon known as 'Acoustic Brainwave Entrainment'. The first article on this was published in *Scientific American* in 1973 by a researcher named Gerald Oster (Oster 1973).

The brainwaves of children with ASD and ADHD are often loosely coordinated and do not come together in a coherent pattern. They are unable to filter out irrelevant information and so cannot get on with what they have been asked to do. In America research studies have shown that neurofeedback can be at least as effective as drugs in alleviating symptoms and producing more relaxed brain patterns. To learn more, go to https://www.centerforbrain.com/neurofeedback/neurofeedback-research/.

Julian, our assistant headteacher, offered to be trained during the summer holidays in the delivery of neurofeedback. Such dedicated staff – aren't our teachers amazing? He was trained in neurofeedback in July 2016. We then purchased the neurofeedback equipment and began offering training to students in spring 2017. The student is able to draw, read or play on their iPad while the brainwave entrainment happens. Parents/carers had to give consent before a student could take part.

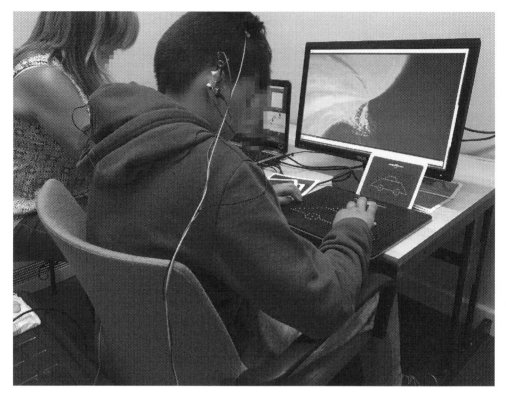

Figure 9.1 Neurofeedback training

The first student we chose had a history of challenging behaviour and staff were already beginning to ask whether our school was the right school for him. He had many challenging behaviour incidences during the week. In fact, he could have between three and five incidences in one day!

He found it impossible to sleep and had done since birth. He had once asked me if he could take a large cardboard box home to see if he would be able to sleep in that – his mind was always on the go. After a week of neurofeedback, staff noticed a difference.

After ten days, his carer came to see me unannounced. She said she just had to come and thank me. For the first time ever, he was sleeping through the night. She was so used to being disturbed by him in the night that she now found herself getting up to watch him sleep. She informed me that he was now able to reason things out rather than hit out.

He went from sometimes having 30 incidences of challenging behaviour per week in school to between one and three incidences per month. In fact, we now noticed these behaviours because they were so rare, and we could usually find the underlying reason for them. Neurofeedback is like going to a gym for your brain. The effects are accumulative over time. Because of his extremely challenging behaviour, his progress using neurofeedback was so noticeable – as can be seen from his behaviour report below.

Behaviour Support Report by BD – HLTA Behaviour Support
3rd July 2017
Report on Jon Doe: Effectiveness of neurofeedback therapy

JD commenced neurofeedback therapy week commencing 15th April; he attends one session on a daily basis. Since attending his behaviour has improved immensely; he is calmer, listens to adults and takes on board reasons as to why things have to happen in such a way. He is happier in himself and appears to be less anxious.

SIMS Behaviour Records for JD since 25th April – a twelve-week period:

- 3rd May fighting on yard (afternoon)
- 15th May verbal abuse to staff (afternoon)
- 6th June assault to staff (afternoon)

Of the above behaviours one incident needed to be logged in the bound and numbered book.*

SIMS behaviours logged in the previous six-week period, (27th February–7th April) before commencing Neuro feedback therapy:

- 3rd March disruptive behaviour (afternoon)
- 6th March assault to staff and pupils (morning)
- 10th March assault to pupil (morning)
- 13th March disruptive behaviour (afternoon)
- 16th March absconded (afternoon)
- 16th March assault to pupil (afternoon)
- 16th March verbal abuse to staff (afternoon)
- 21st March disruptive behaviour (afternoon)
- 21st March assault to pupil (morning)
- 21st March disruptive behaviour (afternoon)
- 22nd March disruptive behaviour (afternoon)
- 28th March assault to staff (morning)
- 28th March disruptive behaviour (morning)

Of the above incidents, six incidents were logged in the bound and numbered book.*

* A bound and numbered book is a central reference record for recording the use of restraint. Information on using restraint can be found at https://www.teamteach.co.uk.

He went onto a secondary special school in 2019 and is doing very well. Ysgol Pen Coch continues to offer neurofeedback to its students.

Neurofeedback has also been proven to support those with dyslexia. Steve, who trained Julian in neurofeedback, told us that his wife, a dyslexic tutor, found that using neurofeedback had a faster effect on improvements with her students than her usual methods.

The psychiatric drugs industry makes millions of pounds every year. In contrast to drugs, once neurofeedback has trained the brain to produce different patterns of electrical communication, no further treatment is necessary. Drugs do not change fundamental brain activity and work only for as long as the patient keeps taking them.

Neurofeedback has been proven to help charge up areas in the brain that are not working and also create new brainwave patterns. The feedback can reinforce selected brainwave patterns while discouraging others. Neurofeedback has no negative side effects.

Here is a link to show how neurofeedback is effective for children: https://vimeo.com/326732410.

Sound support to assist with reading

ARROW is defined as a multisensory teaching/learning system based on the use of the student's own recorded voice, the SelfVoice™, and is used by groups of students work-ing under overt supervision from a tutor. I have used the ARROW machine with students who have dyslexia for many years.

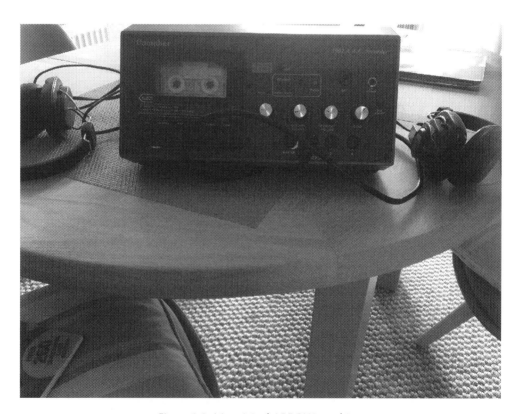

Figure 9.2 My original ARROW machine

I purchased my ARROW machine from Dr Colin Lane in the 1990s when a cassette tape system was used. Dr Lane taught me how to use it with my students at the Gwent Dyslexia Centre. The acronym ARROW stands for aural, read, respond, oral, write.

I found it was able to increase reading and spelling ages in students, and I understand it is still an extremely popular piece of equipment and has changed to accommodate the advances in technology. Future Education, an independent special school in Norwich, receives training in delivering the latest ARROW support to its students in the autumn of 2020. The success is undoubtedly in the student hearing themselves read words correctly, which the machine helps them to do. To receive training and find out more about ARROW, go to https://www.arrowtuition.co.uk/arrow-in-schools. To watch ARROW in action, go to https://www.youtube.com/watch?v=BH1K-KQsjNw.

I vividly recall the sight of a six-foot two-inch biker riding up on my driveway some years ago, with a shaved head (apart from his ponytail), in the hope that the ARROW machine would at last help him to read and write. It did.

Throughout this book we have looked at the way special schools can use music, sound and vibration to deliver a therapeutic curriculum for students to allow them to be in the right frame of mind to learn. Not all students will benefit from every therapy discussed and it is important that assessments are done to match the right therapy to the right student. We will now look at how we can use assessment for music, sound and vibration in a special school.

10 | Assessment

Assessment data is used in many different ways in schools today. It can be used to determine a school's success or failure or indeed the success or failure of an individual member of staff. Being an ex-headteacher of a special school I can see the value in both.

I have found assessment data useful to identify the continual professional development needs of staff members so that they are confident working with children with complex learning needs. I have found that assessment practices rigorously peer-monitored through submission of evidence to special schools' moderation consortiums ensure that teacher judgements in school are in line with best practice in the sector.

The whole point of children being educated in special schools is that their learning is, among other things, idiosyncratic and often non-linear. Comparative data may be meaningful for mainstream schools, but I would question its validity in special education.

The small size of special school cohorts and the nature of their students' learning and progress means that comparisons between year groups cannot easily be made. Progress must be tracked at an individual level to generate meaningful conclusions that support the teaching approaches to be used for that student. CSAM (Connecting Steps Assessment Module, previously called GAP) is a useful data analysis tool for individual schools which I have used. It generates graphs and other charts describing progress for individual children and groups of children in school, across all assessed subjects. It does not compare students in other schools, and although I have used data comparison tools in the past, I have not found them useful enough to warrant the expenditure. CSAM provided me with individualised analysis of progression, and over time generated a progression curve from which future attainment could be projected, and provided a range of ways of displaying this information.

All told, assessment is still an indication of the education that is on offer and a report on the school's use of assessment should be given to the governing body at least once a year. Having first ensured the safety and well-being of the children, the business of any school is that the children make progress in their learning, their skills and understanding. Critical self-analysis of robust assessment data enables a school to evaluate the impact on progress of current working practices, and prompts courses of action to improve learning outcomes. When inspecting schools for Estyn we were always told to look for the impact it made on students' learning.

Summative assessment

Summative assessment is the formal summing up of a pupil's progress that can then be used for purposes ranging from providing information to parents to obtaining qualifications as part of a formal examination course. I have not, as yet, come across a student in a special school taking part in external examinations for music, but it would be essential to ensure that all teachers engaged in making judgements in such a context were working in comparable ways to an agreed set of criteria and standards. There are some students who may benefit from this. I would check first whether they were interested, as sometimes the pressure of exams is not helpful, in contrast to the enjoyment of performing. Derek Paravicini has severe learning difficulties, is blind and autistic. He gave his first concert aged seven and at the age of nine he played with the Royal Philharmonic Pops Orchestra at the Barbican. He enjoys performing.

We would ordinarily use a summative assessment at the end of each term to show whether a student had achieved their IEP targets and at the end of each school year to show whether they had achieved their annual targets, and if they had made progress over the year. What should be taught and therefore assessed to provide a report of a student's musical development whilst in a special school could be controversial to those with a purely music bias.

- The therapist in music would provide an assessment report on every student she had worked with over the year, but that report might not just be about music progression and would be dependent upon goals set by the class teacher, sometimes to do with behaviour.
- The therapist in music would also routinely report on a child's progress to parents in time for an annual review of their child's progress.
- The therapist would adopt manageable recording procedures that enable them to keep track of each student's learning, without feeling obliged to record everything.
- The therapist would be able to communicate effectively with each student.
- There would be manageable expectations of the therapist to report at intervals to the class teacher on the students for whom they have a responsibility.
- It is important that class teachers act in a considered way on the formative and summative assessments received from therapists (rather than simply filing them away).
- The class teacher would provide a report on the students' response and involvement during transitional music times, which happen throughout the school day. It is up to the class teacher to monitor this.
- Therapists leading other sessions that involve vibration, sound or music would report individually to class teachers regarding these, but it would be up to the class teacher to specify what they wish the therapist to report on. It may be that these sessions are just the vehicles for helping a student deal with their emotions (PHSE), their movement (PE), their communication (literacy), etc.

Formative assessment

Formative assessment is often daily assessment providing information to take learning forward. It is a central part of pedagogy and essential daily practice in a special school setting.

As a special school headteacher of students primarily with profound or severe learning difficulties and with secondary diagnosis of autism, ADHD and other complex differences, my concern was for most of the year taken up with formative assessment and how we could enable our students to be in the right frame of mind to learn in the first place. Also, to help our students to have a better quality of life, develop life skills and assist them in any subject they showed particular interest in, such as music. This formative assessment would then feed into the summative assessments which, in turn, provided us with information on target setting to take learning forward the following year.

It makes sense to assess a student so that we may help them develop their musical skills and creativity whilst also assessing the impact that sound, music and vibration have on their overall development and their health and well-being. It also shows that you value that subject and the part it plays in the school curriculum.

Assessment tools and frameworks

There are music assessment tools and frameworks available online and there is a lot of free guidance online for assessing students in their musical ability such as the excellent site for the Sounds of Intent (SOI) Framework (see Section 7 of the Appendix). SOI enhances the reliability and validity of the assessment of musical ability.

The Engagement Model (2020) (see Section 9 of the Appendix) is the English guidance for students with SEND and has taken over six years from the release of their new primary curriculum for the DfE to produce. It is not an assessment tool on its own and should be used alongside a school's assessment system. An example of a school's assessment policy is included in chapter 13.

The Engagement Model has been written for students performing at P levels 1–4 (see Section 20 of the Appendix) and is not subject-specific. The updated Routes for Learning (RfL) Framework (see Section 8 of the Appendix) are also useful tools for students not engaged in subject specific study. The Routes for Learning materials support schools in assessing the early communication and cognitive skills of learners with profound and multiple learning difficulties (PMLD). The Quest for Learning Model (see Section 10 of the Appendix) is used in Ireland and is based on the RfL model. B Squared and other commercial assessment packages are also available, and these can be subject-specific, but you pay for them. A skills ladder for music, sound and vibration and linked to the P levels can be found in chapter 13 if you wish to adapt and use it for free in your school.

I feel that RfL and the Engagement Model are more generalised assessment tools that encompass the use of sound, music and vibration but that SOI is specifically for the assessment of musical development and they are all free.

Both RfL and SOI have a visual map that can be used as a classroom poster as observation support for staff, including supply staff, temporary staff and volunteers. They are easy to read, but I would suggest that the class teacher ensures their staff have a good understanding of the maps and that they are regularly referred to during class staff team meetings.

Learning development is not linear, and these maps allow staff to follow the steps students take rather than direct students towards steps that their sensory or physical disabilities prevent them from achieving and thereby causing an impasse.

Assessment programmes

There are some assessment programmes for the older student such as the ASDAN Creative Arts module, which encourages students to learn to play an instrument, and they are then assessed according to specific criteria before a certificate is awarded. ASDAN is a charitable social enterprise whose mission is to create the opportunity for learners to achieve personal and social development through a structured programme of awards and qualifications. I have used ASDAN in schools where the students were old enough to follow the programmes of study. It is fantastic. ASDAN.org.uk tells of a student who was a school refuser and says:

> I am now attending school full time studying English, Maths and music. I am currently passing all of them, with a B- in English and an A in music. . . . I have spoken to groups of adults that I didn't know, to tell them about how ASDAN has helped me. . . . Because of the comforting place of ASDAN, I no longer feel like I want to die.

There are other assessments such as the ABRSM, but I have never had a student in a special school capable of taking their assessments, which usually require a good level of reading ability. There is also BTech creatives, but it is equivalent to GCSE work. Again I personally have no experience of students who have been able to undertake BTech modules or GCSEs in a special school for students with SLD or PMLD. However, I am confident that if a student attending a special school was capable, then staff would assist in any way to help that student achieve qualifications.

Some things to bear in mind

- When assessing any student, it is always more productive to focus on the positives rather than the negatives, and so it is true for students with severe or profound learning difficulties – focus on their abilities rather than disabilities.
- It is important to involve family and professionals in a student's education and health plan (EHP)/individual development plan (IDP)/individual education plan (IEP) in the assessment process where possible so that better learning opportunities are enabled through collaboration.
- Keeping accurate records of therapies /programmes/sessions undertaken and the student's reaction/engagement/communication provides evidence of progression/regression and is extremely important when monitoring, reflecting on and sharing the needs of the student.
- Formative assessment informs everyone concerned on what steps to take next to ensure that the student is enjoying the learning process.
- It would be wrong for any student, in spite of their learning ability or disability, to attend a school where there is no regard for their development, and so assessment is essential for all students.
- Sometimes the learning development of a student with severe health problems might be assisting that student to manage those health problems. All schools should be concerned with preparing students for their own adulthood and the learning goals should reflect that.

* Assessment should not be about making things into a testing or exam-like situation so that the student dreads the activity or is made to feel apprehensive. It is something that should be undertaken with calm confidence by the assessor.
* If you are new to assessing a student with PMLD or SLD and you feel there is no obvious response, try videoing the assessment activity to review later with colleagues.
* Remember that learners may respond more to a familiar face.

Please see the recording and assessment templates in chapter 13 which may help you to promote consistency throughout a school.

Self-assessment and peer-assessment

Self-assessment and peer-assessment has been extremely popular with many of my students over the years, and the well-known traffic lights system has been used where students give themselves a red if they felt they needed a lot of support, yellow if they had some help, and green if they found the task easy. This kind of system can easily be applied to peer assessment. Two stars and a wish is a system that has to be monitored carefully, as I have reviewed students' books where the same wishes were written several times by the teacher immediately after each other.

These kinds of assessment can be used for assessing music development or for the targets associated with a session that includes music. I include templates in chapter 13. Peer assessment and guidance from staff on how we can assess others' performance, given their conditions and restrictions, are essential if peers are to become the supportive human beings we would wish for in our society, and not judgemental harridans.

An assessment policy is provided in chapter 13 for you to adapt and use if you wish.

In the next chapter we will consider the part parents and carers can play in ensuring that they get the best education for their children attending a special school.

11 Parents and carers

The most important people in a child's life are their parents or carers. Parents and carers can have a very positive role to play in their children's education. Parents do not choose to have a child with severe or profound health needs and learning difficulties. Carers do choose.

It is sometimes difficult for a parent or carer with a child who has special needs to find the strength to ensure that their child has the very best of the education that is on offer. Their time is often taken up with caring for their child's health and medical needs.

Attending meetings

Imagine that you have been asked to attend a meeting regarding your child's individual education plan. You know it is vital that you get the best education for your child and you want to be fully informed about what is available, but your child has not slept through the night due to their condition, and so you too have not slept. You attend a meeting where you are surrounded by professionals who are there to help you decide what kind of education is best for your child, and you are tired. How can special schools help parents in these situations?

Often the parents of a child with special needs have health support, social service support or local authority support who will point them in the right direction or even accompany them to meetings if asked. In fact, SEN Reg 9 requires the local authority to consider whether the parents or student requires advice or support. The assessment is carried out by the local authority, but health, social services and education have important parts to play both practically and financially. Sometimes parents find these multi-disciplinary meetings of these services coming together overwhelming and do ask schools for advice.

Supporting parents and section G

As a headteacher I have been asked by concerned parents for advice. I would advise parents/carers that they ask the people who have arranged the meeting to give them an agenda and the necessary information beforehand so that they can go to the meeting prepared. I would inform them, if asked, that the most important part, from an educational perspective, of England's health-care plan, after the type of school, is section G, which is where parents or carers can ask for specific therapies that they feel their child would benefit from. I would encourage parents/carers to visit the school website to see what is on offer.

If a parent knows or thinks that their child benefits from music, then they could ask for therapeutic music to be included on his or her timetable. If a parent feels vibro-acoustic therapy or sound therapy could help, the time to ask for them is during this meeting. If the parents live in Wales, then they would need to mention the therapies they want during the 'How to Support' section of the meeting and insist it is written into the Action Plan. Whichever country you live in there will be an education plan that purports to support a child through school.

If a parent feels that any other of the therapies I have written about in this book would help their child, then this meeting is when parents get the opportunity to ask for it to be included. Of course, the schools in their authority may not provide these, but there is a saying: 'if you do not ask you do not get'. I have attended many, many annual reviews over the years and I could count on just one hand the number of students who had a specific therapy referred to on their statement (which meant that that therapy had to be provided by the school). Those parents were either in the field of education themselves and knew what was available or they had done their research. Section 37(1) of the Children and Families Act states that 'once an EHC plan has been prepared, it must maintain the plan'. This is the same for any education plan and parents have a right to complain if their child's needs are not being met. It is always good when parents and schools can work together to ensure that children's needs are being met. The Investors in Families (IIF) award is a quality mark that recognises the work that schools undertake with families to help ensure the needs of children and young people attending school are being met.

It is my experience as a special school senior manager and as a headteacher that as a rule parents and carers only ever want what they believe is best for the children they care for. Parents and carers know their children better than anyone. The best chair of governors I ever had was a parent of one of our students who had PMLD. It is sometimes very difficult as a parent of a child with special needs to find the time to become involved in school life. Their time is so often taken up with many healthcare meetings and sometimes social care meetings and they need respite time when they know that their child is being well cared for and educated in school. Yet there are many advantages to becoming fully involved in the school life of a child. It is important that parents and carers attend the regular parent evenings that a school provides as well as the once a year annual review of the student's EHC or individual development plan to support both their educational and well-being needs whilst the student attends the school, which could be for a number of years. These meetings allow parents to find out how their children are progressing and whether any particular therapy could aid that progress. It is the school's responsibility to provide a language translator at those meetings if one is required.

Communication

In a special school most students would have a home school diary that travels back and forth so that parents and school staff can update each other daily on the students' needs and progress and communicate effectively. Parent apps are now popular and easily connect parents to the school via the phone making it easy to pay for school meals etc.

When parents take an active interest in their child's time in school, they get to know what is available, they can experience these things for themselves and ensure that their child and other people's children get every opportunity that's available to them. Parent governors get the opportunity to become more involved in their child's therapies and education by going on governor learning walks and joining committees that influence the school's development. I always found parent governors to be the most supportive governors when it came to introducing an innovative therapy into the school. Every year schools in Wales provide a governor report to parents. It is no longer statutory to do so in England.

Parent partnership

It is useful for special school parents to have a parent partnership which allows parents to attend sessions in school where they can learn singing and signing for themselves, where they can find out about the therapies on offer and perhaps experience them for themselves so that they have a better understanding of what happens during a session. One of my higher-level teaching assistants (HLTA) ran our parent partnership workshops and events for us and it was well attended by parents desperate to see how they could help their children at home as well as understand what was available to their child in school. Parents have been able to try all the therapies mentioned in this book. Family events happened regularly in school time and still do at that school, and music often has a big part to play in these. Sometimes a school has the budget for a family liaison officer who will take over the running of parent partnership events and provide support to the family. Our school was able to finance this for a couple of years. Family liaison support can include helping parents to fill in complex forms, attend reviews with them and accompany them on other meetings that the headteacher gives approval for. The liaison officer can signpost parents or carers to useful organisations and develop links with these organisations so that the school can further support families.

School and family events include music sessions, concerts, assemblies and curriculum/therapy conferences. We held international conferences on therapeutic interventions and parents and carers volunteered to speak out at these conferences about the benefits these therapies had had on their children.

If the school has a hydrotherapy pool it may be useful to start up a pre-school 'Bubbles' group for babies and toddlers who have been diagnosed by physiotherapists as benefiting from the use of a hydrotherapy pool. I was able to introduce this into the school. Soothing, calming music is always used during these sessions and many of the babies and toddlers who attended the sessions eventually attended our school full time and found the transition easier as a result. The pool session was always followed by coffee and a chat.

PTA

A parent teacher association (PTA) is also important and we found that ours fundraised for many of the therapies we introduced because they had seen first-hand the effects on their children. These parent support groups are a great support to each other. They often have an online presence so that they can be easily and cheaply contacted. Sometimes parents can help a PTA in other ways, such as approaching local businesses for raffle prizes and 'behind the scenes' support that is equally valuable. Our PTA helped raise funds to ensure our holiday club – which ran for five of the six weeks of summer recess – continued, and they purchased equipment for the club that could also be used to improve school facilities for all.

When you consider the needs of our students, it was very important for our staff and the parents that the students were able to continue to access the facilities and a structured routine if it was needed. The holiday club was always full, so that probably speaks for itself. Music played a big part in the holiday club, and where possible transitional music was still played, so that when school resumed in the autumn term the transition to full-time education was not so daunting for the students. There are many websites that can offer support to schools wishing to set up a parents' association or even a parent–teacher association. One such site is www. parentkind.org.uk.

It is worth remembering that if you as a member of the school staff have an online presence, then you possibly will be contacted online by parents for advice. You then have to decide if you wish to limit who can contact you. I had and still have an online presence and was contacted by parents via my Twitter account, and I can honestly say I never minded. Every parent deserves to feel listened to and valued. There is a line between ensuring your views as a parent are heard and demanding that your views are the only views that matter. I said earlier that, as a rule, parents only ever want what they perceive to be best for their children, but it is also worth saying that, as a rule, schools only ever want what is best for their students' education and well-being.

Our school also had a Twitter account, as do most schools today. Twitter can show parents what their children had been up to during the day. Twitter will allow you to link a video so that if parents or carers have missed a child's concert, they can watch it online or on their phone. Keep in mind that you need parent permission beforehand for any photos or videos that you show.

School website

The traditional way of keeping parents informed in the past was through a school prospectus. These are still useful documents for showcasing what a school provides for its students and are still produced by many schools to hand out to prospective parents. They have now been superseded by the school website, which should have links to most information that an interested parent or carer might need.

A school website will show parents, carers and visitors to the site everything that the school offers and should contain important policies and information so that they can keep up to date. It will also contain all information on the therapies and curriculum on offer by the school. I found that many parents used our website to find out about the therapies, and then contacted us to ask that their children accessed the therapies they had prioritised. Our school website also had a separate parent/carer/student section that only they could log into. This contained annual reviews, individual education plans, individual behaviour plans, etc. Although copies of these would be sent home, it was important for me that parents could download a spare copy if they needed to. The section also contained many photos of their child, as it was cheaper to put them onto the website than print off copies daily to send home. If parents chose to print off and share a picture of their child enjoying any of the therapies mentioned in this book with families and friends, that was up to them.

Homeschooling

Sometimes special school students need to be homeschooled for a time. Perhaps they have been in hospital and are recovering, for instance. A member of staff would need to be assigned to supporting that child in the home. A policy is necessary to protect everyone involved. Some students would return to school in stages, perhaps returning for hydrotherapy sessions and therapeutic music sessions or vibro-acoustic sessions. A plan is drawn up between home and school and reviewed regularly. Due to most families being able to access the internet, a lot of interactive experiences can now be posted on a school website for students to join in from home. This works especially well for the music curriculum.

In a school where you have many students with PMLD, you may have to attend funerals of some of these students, and music has, in my experience, played a big part where schools can be a support to families (if families wish it). Remembrance services are often helpful for the rest of the students, and again music is a therapeutic factor to be borne in mind when planning such a service. I remember every funeral and remembrance service I attended because of the music that was played.

The year 2020 has been particularly challenging for families of children with special needs due to the coronavirus pandemic, and we will look at these effects on the delivery of music and therapeutic interventions. It is safe to say that the partnership between home and school has never been more important.

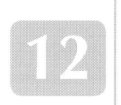

The effects of the coronavirus pandemic on the delivery of music and therapeutic interventions in special schools

During the coronavirus pandemic most children were homeschooled unless the family had members who were key workers. I had contact with special schools during this time and supported a couple of schools through Team and Zoom meetings. I also provided links to useful sites for parents: www.linkedin.com/pulse/free-learning-home-during-corona-virus-threat-ange-anderson/.

I remained in contact with many schools that I have worked alongside in the past and I know that they fully supported their students during this time. This meant for some staff working in school with key workers' children and working online with the rest of the students. Music continued to play a big part in students' education. If you were to visit most special schools' websites during that time you would have seen links to singing and signing videos, dancing to music videos and links to online yoga, and therapeutic and technological music. Students could still benefit from meditation and mindfulness via online links established by the schools. Throughout this book I refer to these online links. The added bonus is that now all those schools have these links for parents to access in the future when needed. There is always a silver lining.

What are the best ways for schools and parents to work together during this time of uncertainty to ensure that students' needs are being met? The assistant director for Peterborough and Cambridgeshire is Toni Bailey. He is responsible for SEND and inclusion and he told me:

> We have seen an impact on the ability for schools to deliver the whole of the EHC plan provision over the course of the pandemic, although in England there was a period of 'easements' on the duty to provide elements of the EHC plan allowing local authorities (LAs) to use their 'best endeavours' in order to meet the duties. It has been hugely challenging to ensure that children get access to all of the services they need. This has had a tremendous impact particularly on families, who have been managing our most complex children at home for many months.

The easements to legislation came to an end in September 2020 and this has left local authorities with the duty to provide the full EHC plan, including any social care or health needs/therapies outlined. This has presented some significant challenges, as the DfE guidance and the NHS England guidance have not always been aligned.

At Peterborough and Cambridgeshire they have been successfully managing to work with colleagues in health to consider the differences in guidance, and where it is deemed necessary to interact face to face (in person) to get the required outcome, therapy services are delivered in person, utilising the appropriate risk assessment and personal protective equipment (PPE). Toni says:

> In the main this has been really successful and partnership working with parent forums has been key in managing the expectations of parents and young people. I think we have managed to find the right balance and we do have therapy services going into schools regularly, but it is reduced and our ability to provide remote options that can be effective has massively improved, with some young people and families' feedback outlining how they prefer the remote approach (especially with our ASC community). This means we need to review our long-term approaches and learn from the positives from the last 6 months. There are still challenges ahead, but we have to embrace the possibility that a different mode of delivery may have to be the new standard if we are to do what we can to reduce the spread of Covid-19, which remains a priority.

I believe that the most difficult part of the pandemic for students was not having access to individual hands-on therapies. I believe that parents and carers of students with PMLD and those students themselves possibly suffered more than most. This is because a special school has such amazing facilities these days and students can be free of their wheelchairs for a good part of the day and have appropriate therapeutic input from trained staff.

In the autumn of 2020 students returned to school unless they needed to self-isolate at home or required shielding. Remote education continued for these students. I have spoken to many headteachers during the pandemic and also during the first month of those students being able to return to school. All headteachers agree that this has been a very difficult period for parents, and headteachers have tried their very best to support parents and students during this time. I am reliably informed that headteachers have worked 12-hour days seven days a week throughout the lockdown and continued to do so when schools reopened in order to be fully versed on every Covid update, as well as produce up-to-date risk assessments for every student so that PPE was personalised (PPE can be basic, from simple face coverings to including aprons and gloves, to the full surgical kit when dealing with gastrostomy tubing, for instance).

Headteachers have praised the dedication of their staff in meeting the needs of students both in school and those educated at home under school direction. As Chris Britten, head of Ysgol Y Deri in Penarth (the largest special school in Great Britain and subject of a BBC documentary in September 2020: www.bbc.co.uk/programmes/p08qj7yx), told me:

> School staff have to be looked after so that they are there to look after the children. One member of staff affected by the virus can impact on a lot of the students. As a school we offer both in-person and remote learning. Currently our technician has tested positive and so the senior leadership team along with the multi-disciplinary team will have an online meeting to discuss current guidelines already in practice and new risks and act accordingly. We have to keep our staff safe as well as keep our students safe.

He likened it to the needle on a record player. If you take care of that needle, then all records play well.

I spoke to both Noel Fitzgerald, head of Ysgol Pen Coch, and Julian Lewis, assistant head of Ysgol Pen Coch. Noel told me, 'We have physios and SALT back in school but in a carefully managed way. They are both using the school hall at present as we are unable to use if for lunch or any other activities due to the restrictions.'

Julian added, 'Staff take students to the hall, rather than them dropping into class to collect them, as they did in the past. It's all about protecting the class bubble where possible.'

He continued: 'So we had to change home time procedures for minibuses, use of playground – only one class out at a time, lunches taken in class, no community trips'.

Noel has found music the easiest subject to deliver throughout the crisis, and now that staff and pupils are back in school, music plays as important a part as ever in transition times. He went on to tell me:

> We are using the other therapy rooms but are having to tightly timetable sessions for 'bubbles' of pupils and have factored in cleaning time in between. Hydrotherapy has continued as it is a relatively safe activity given the amount of bug killing chemicals in the pool. Rebound therapy is one we haven't run up to now – the cleaning of the trampoline and safe use for staff/ pupils is one which I am hoping to come up with a solution for, so it can return after half term.

Julian added that some therapies continue (without some resources). For instance, soft play continues without the ball pool, as it would be too time consuming to clean the plastic balls after every session. He confirmed that hydrotherapy was happening for students in the school but that all those students from other schools, who would benefit from being out of their wheelchairs and free in the pool, cannot attend due to the restrictions.

Julian told me that the hands-on therapies obviously could not continue so they have been postponed for now. These include neurofeedback, some play therapy involving small toy parts, magic therapy and auditory integration therapy.

Noel is trying to encourage therapy sessions within the class delivered by the class team rather than peripatetic staff and has engaged on sharing good practice between experienced therapy-trained staff to support other staff to deliver this. This means they can access therapies while safely remaining in their class bubble with their class staff team.

Julian told me that some students have shown a dip in attainment or behaviour which the senior management team believe can be linked to time away from school, but overall they don't believe that there has been any negative behaviour that they can link directly to any anxiety arising to the lockdown. 'That's not to say there isn't but there is nothing that we can specifically associate it with.'

Noel added,

> On the whole the children have been very happy to be back and have just got on with school. A couple of children and staff have tested negative following concerns about temperature, but we are following guidance regarding that to the letter.

Donna Roberts, head of Ysgol Hafod Lon in Penrhyndeudraeth, told me:

> Being in school at this time is tough, staff shortages due to self-isolation and also just general illness is a huge struggle, but staff are anxious and at times overwhelmed by the responsibility and restrictions. We are continuing with all therapies except for hydrotherapy at the moment but staff wearing PPE and cleaning in between each session means less time for the pupils to receive the actual therapy.

Andreas Huws, head of Ysgol Y Bont on the island of Anglesey, has found it difficult to get the external therapy services such as the physiotherapy team and the speech and language team to visit the island school and a lot of partnership work has initially been done via Team and Skype meetings, though he is applying pressure to have this extended, as 'I really want them on the shop floor assessing/interacting/advising'.

Jonathan Morgan, head of Ysgol Gogarth in Llandudno, told me:

> We have had to adapt and change some of our practice and the biggest change is that we cannot give as much therapeutic intervention to some pupils as we would like. This is mostly because of restrictions around 'bubbles' and trying to minimise the spread of infection when we do have a positive case in the school (staff or pupil). At the same time, we have recognised that attending school without some essential therapies would be detrimental to some children's well-being and future progress. Currently we are continuing to do some hands-on physio despite health not currently providing it. We are reopening the hydrotherapy pool to certain 'bubbles'. We are still allowing music and have a music therapist and art therapy student in school every week. School would be very boring without the important therapies for our most vulnerable learners.

Rhona O'Neil, head of Ysgol Tir Morfa in Rhyl, has used the time to ensure staff therapy training during the lockdown and has continued to deliver music in all its forms via the internet, as have all of the schools I have been able to speak to. It just goes to show that music is a subject than can still be delivered by a special school and enjoyed by its students even during a lockdown.

13 Resources and support

In this book you will have seen how different therapeutic interventions can transform the lives and enhance the learning capabilities of students. You will have seen how important it is not only to use transitional music but also to have a policy as a fundamental guideline for all staff on desired outcomes. In this chapter you will find the resources and policies mentioned throughout the book. I have included these free resources so that you do not have to start from scratch as I did. Please feel free to photocopy and adapt to suit your school.

Resource 13.1 Assessment, recording and reporting policy
Appendix 1 Assessment file contents
Resource 13.2 Eye Gaze policy
Resource 13.3 Hydrotherapy policy
Resource 13.4 Meditation and mindfulness policy
Resource 13.5 Singing and signing policy
Resource 13.6 Tacpac policy
Resource 13.7 Therapeutic music policy
Resource 13.8 Transitional music policy
Resource 13.9 Vibro-acoustic therapy policy
Resource 13.10 Vibro-acoustic therapy impact report for governors – autumn term
Resource 13.11 Free music resources and support
Resource 13.12 Therapeutic music report for parents
Table 13.1 Soundbeam targets
Table 13.2 POPAT AIT research data
Table 13.3 Risk assessments
Table 13.4 Music, sound and vibrations skills ladder
Table 13.5 Vibro-acoustic therapy (VAT) screening form
Table 13.6 Visual analogue scale

Resource 13.1 Assessment, recording and reporting policy

Date:

Assessment of pupils' needs and abilities, recording their achievements and experiences, and reporting these to parents and other professionals is central to the provision of education at our school. This is primarily the responsibility of teachers, with input from support staff where appropriate. The aim of recording and assessment is to give a clear picture of where the pupil is now and to inform future planning. At classroom level, particularly, there is little intrinsic value in recording information as an end in itself but rather it is important to view the whole continuous process of planning, recording and evaluating as a means of meeting pupils' needs more effectively and of monitoring progress accurately.

All records relating to any individual pupil are accessible to her/his parents on request and to professionals working within the school as appropriate, but are regarded as confidential documents. From time to time professionals external to the school may have access to records for a specific purpose. Parents can also access many confidential documents relating to their child, e.g. IEP targets and behaviour plans via a secure login on the school website. Students and volunteers do not have direct access to records but may request specific information related to their studies from the member of staff supervising their placement. No documents relating to individual pupils may be photocopied for use outside the school without permission of the headteacher.

Classroom assessment and recording

Teaching plans

Medium-term plans give an outline of the skills to be covered in each subject area. Weekly teaching plans are drawn from these.

Annual targets and individual education plans

Individual annual targets are set for each academic year, using the Engagement Model or Routes for Learning (RfL) assessment tools, and B Squared. In some instances, this may incorporate another tool, such as the Sounds of Intent (SOI) framework. Sounds of Intent is an assessment framework for those making music with children and young people with learning difficulties (ranging from PMLD to SLD to autism). Sounds of Intent is designed to help teachers and parents relate what they observe in music sessions with a child into more concrete statements/levels.

This process involves parents/carers in the form of a parents' evening and as part of the annual review process, as well as pupils, wherever possible. These are then broken down into termly IEP targets for an individual pupil.

Pupils are also set termly IEP targets, one each taken from the Literacy, Numeracy and Digital Competence Frameworks. The school follows a regular pattern of target setting from certain strands/

elements of the Literacy and Numeracy Frameworks, which follows the scheme of a Moderation Consortium. This facilitates the school's participation in the consortium for moderation purposes.

IEP sheets for the past three terms as well as annual targets for the past two years are kept in the pupil's assessment file. Earlier IEPs and annual targets are filed in the pupil's confidential files, which are kept in a secure cabinet in the office. Progress against annual targets is collated at the end of the summer term.

Individual subject learning outcomes

For pupils in Foundation Phase and Key Stage 2 pupil progress in all other subject areas is assessed against the Routes for Learning, Foundation Phase Footsteps and the Foundation Phase Framework curriculum skills documents.

Behaviour records

Where a child is identified as having challenging behaviours, a behaviour plan will be written. Where it is anticipated that such a pupil may require physical intervention as part of the behaviour management strategies that are supportive of them, a positive handling plan will be written to be read in conjunction with the individual behaviour plan. Copies will be kept in the class 'Keeping Safe' folder with additional copies held by the midday supervisor's coordinator and the behaviour coordinator. Behaviour frequency charts and/or antecedent behaviour consequence (ABC) charts may be used for analysis of patterns in behaviour and response to intervention. Incidents involving extremes of behaviour are recorded on SIMS, in addition to any accident/near miss reporting required. Extreme behaviours that have resulted in restraint of the pupil (permitted for their own safety, the safety of others, the prevention of damage to school property or prevention of criminal acts) are recorded in the Bound and Numbered Book, following the Team Teach procedure. Specific behaviour targets may be set as part of IEPs for some pupils as appropriate.

Inclusion folders

Where pupils are involved in regular integration in mainstream school, their responses and achievement are recorded in integration files. These are individual or group files depending on the nature of the integration project. Arranging recording/observations is the responsibility of the class teacher sending the pupil to an inclusion activity. They will have to provide the TA who takes the child with the relevant targets and guidance to enable them to do the recording. The mainstream class teacher providing the inclusion opportunity may also be invited to record comments.

Administrative records

Central file

Each pupil has a central file located in the school office. This contains background referral information, correspondence with external agencies, correspondence with parents, reports from professionals such as psychologists, copies of annual reviews and annual reports and the school copy of the child's Statement of Special Educational Need. These files are available for class teachers, who should sign them out when required, but they are not to be taken from the school premises.

Pupil information file

Data checking sheets are kept in this file in the school office and provide a quick reference when addresses or emergency contact numbers are required.

Attendance records

It is a legal responsibility for the class teacher to keep and maintain an accurate register of pupils in their class. The school uses the SIMS system to enable teachers to do so. Teachers must use the correct presence, lateness and absence codes to enable a genuine picture of a child's attendance to be given so that patterns of poor attendance can be spotted, reasons investigated (e.g. lateness may be because of their transport route, not because the family is not ready on time), constructive solutions sought, and if necessary support from the Education Welfare Officer called in. Attendance is reported to parents in the annual review. Staff should initiate action regarding unauthorised absences in line with the school's pupil attendance policy.

Pupil records on SIMS system

Basic information about pupils is kept on the SIMS data system. The school secretary is responsible for maintaining this information in an up to date form. Information kept is supplied by parents/carers, usually on admission to the school. Staff who become aware of subsequent changes should inform the school secretary. This information is supplied to the local authority (LA) and government through statutory census returns. Each pupil has a unique pupil number (UPN) for this process. Data held and exchanged in this way complies with data protection legislation. All pupil and school data are held and used in accordance with the general data protection regulations.

Medical records

Medical records are kept in a locked filing cabinet in the nurse's room to which only the school nurse has access. These are updated regularly by the school nurse.

Records for regular medication and emergency medication are kept in the nurse's room. These are filled in by the school nurse or by those with delegated responsibility for administering the medication.

Transport information

The school secretary maintains a list relating to which contractors are responsible for transporting which pupils.

Early years assessment

Foundation Stage profile assessments

In line with government and county requirements, children who are entering the Foundation Stage are assessed using the Foundation Stage profile document. The assessment is kept in the pupils' assessment files as evidence. A school-devised summary of the assessment is recorded and kept on the school server. This forms a starting point from which to evaluate an individual's future progress and facilitates group comparisons with pupils in other years and from other schools.

It is also recognised that all children entering the nursery have been referred by early years professionals as having some degree of developmental delay or special educational need. In most cases background information including developmental and normative data has been made available by these professionals to both parents and school staff.

The Foundation Stage profile assessment undertaken is in four main areas of the pre-school curriculum – language, literacy and communication, mathematical development, personal and social development, and physical development. Assessment is based on classroom observations during the first six weeks of entering the Foundation Department.

End of Key Stage assessment

All schools have a statutory obligation to assess the level of achievement of individual pupils at the end of the Foundation Stage (Year 2) and end of Key Stage 2 (Year 6). This information is reported to the government during national data collection each May. The current internal school requirements are as follows:

Foundation Department

Teacher assessment – subject outcome level for:

* Language, literacy and communication
* Mathematical development
* Personal and social development
* Physical development

Tests/tasks (if not disapplied):

* Literacy
* Numeracy

Pupils' achievements are assessed against the Foundation Phase and KS2 Curriculum Outcome Statement. From 2018 Year 2 pupils will be assessed using the Foundation Phase

Profile document. This will demonstrate progress from entry into the Foundation Phase to the end of Year 2.

Key Stage 2

Teacher assessment – subject outcome level for:

* English
* Welsh
* Mathematics
* Science

Tests/tasks (if not disapplied):

* Literacy
* Numeracy

Teacher assessment

The assessment of individual achievements is an integral feature of the work of the school. Teachers evaluate individual annual and IEP targets; evidence skills gained each term and summarise these achievements in end of year reports. For many of our pupils it is not appropriate to measure progress in terms of National Curriculum levels of achievement. The pre-levels (known as P levels/scales – see Section 20 of the Appendix) specified in national guidance for target setting in special schools will be used to supplement ongoing teacher assessment. These will be averaged and converted as appropriate to both Foundation and KS2 outcomes for the purposes of National Data Collection every May. These assessments will be carried out in the spring term of the appropriate year where pupils' work will be moderated by Foundation teachers to determine end of Foundation outcomes and KS2 teachers to determine KS2 outcomes.

Literacy and Numeracy Framework, and Digital Competence Framework

Teachers along with input from teaching assistants assess pupils against the statements within the Literacy and Numeracy Framework (LNF) to determine pupils' abilities and to plan the next steps in their learning. A rolling programme of LNF strands to be targeted throughout the school corresponds to the moderation focuses within the moderation network. This ensures coverage of the LNF to raise the standards in all areas of literacy and numeracy throughout the school. Planning formats have also been adapted to ensure the coverage of LNF skills within all subject areas taught. Parents also receive information regarding pupils' strengths and areas for development within literacy and numeracy in the form of a short narrative statement as part of pupils' end of year reports which also details areas for development.

A Digital Competence Framework was introduced with a robust assessment for this.

National literacy and numeracy tests

Due to the severe and profound learning difficulties of our pupils it is likely in most if not all cases that the national tests will be inaccessible even with modification and developmentally entirely inappropriate to their needs. All such children will be disapplied from the national tests using the procedure currently in force in the region.

Teachers will use their professional judgement to assess whether a child in their class will benefit from taking either the tests designed for that child's chronological age group, or a test taken from a lower chronological age group. Any child taking a test or tests for a lower age group must also be disapplied from the national tests, which assess according to chronological age. A child may take one, two or all three tests and be disapplied from the others.

Teachers putting children forward to sit national tests for the chronological age group must administer the tests in accordance with all government guidance provided, observing the time frame required (typically a week in early May). Their papers must be sent to the government for marking and analysis.

Children who take a test or tests from a lower age group may do so outside the test window. Their papers provide information for internal use in school and do not need to be sent to the government.

Work evidence

Teachers will maintain an assessment folder for each child in their class. The assessment folder must contain a specified range of evidence, as detailed in Appendix 1.

In class assessment procedures

Formal assessment

The management of formal assessment procedures at Stage 5 of the code of practice for pupils with SEN is the responsibility of the local education authority and is usually undertaken as pupils approach statutory school age. Several professionals are involved in this process. Class teachers are responsible for submitting information required by the LA from the school. The educational psychologist is also likely to meet and observe the child in school currently.

Assessment tools

The school uses a range of assessment tools depending on the needs of the child concerned – see table overleaf. Teachers use their professional judgement to decide which assessment tool best meets the needs of any given child in their class. Teachers must update the assessment profiles towards the end of each term, providing the data required for assessment analysis within school.

Condition	PMLD	SLD	Autism
Assessment tool in use 2018–2019	Routes for Learning	B Squared Connecting Steps: P levels/National Curriculum levels	B Squared Connecting Steps: Autism Progress
Target headings	My Communication	English	Communication
	My Thinking	Maths	Flexibility of Thought
	My Care and Independence	PHSE	Social Interaction
			Emotional Regulation
	Computing	Computing	Computing
Framework targets	Literacy	Literacy	Literacy
	Numeracy	Numeracy	Numeracy
	Digital Competence	Digital Competence	Digital Competence
Additional areas assessed, but targets not set	PE Language (e.g. Welsh) (using Connecting Steps P levels/National Curriculum levels) Music (Using SOE Framework)		

It is recognised that learners with PMLD learn in highly idiosyncratic ways and typically find generalisation and retention challenging. Teachers at our school make use of an eight-point scale to indicate the pupils' degree of mastery of the target:

1. Passive or rejection
2. Encounter
3. Awareness
4. Attention and response
5. Engagement
6. Participation
7. Initiation
8. Imitation

(There is also now a five-point scale from the Engagement Model, 2020.)

Until such time as the pupil achieves imitation, the teacher will revisit the target as necessary with the pupil to enable them to develop their competency in it. It will not be appropriate for a teacher to continually set the same target until imitation is reached. Rather they will plan for a rich curriculum experience in the usual way and re-set the target at an appropriate future point.

CSAM

Connecting Steps Assessment Module is the data analysis package that supports assessment tracking in any of the B Squared stable of assessment tools. CSAM enables school to monitor progress of all children, groups of children and individual children in the school. Support needs can begin to be identified through this data, e.g. any communication difficulties, beneficial therapies, or other classroom intervention.

CSAM is a stand-alone analysis tool: it does not compare an individual's results against any supposed sector norm. We believe this is robust and sufficient when looking at the attainment and achievement of children with SEN as their learning is individual and typically non-linear. Comparing one child with SLD or autism to another supposedly equivalent child is not the same as looking at cohorts of neurotypical children.

Likewise, school no longer sets end of phase or Key Stage targets for children as such predictions are based on inherently linear models of progression that do not apply to our children.

These considerations follow the recommendations of the Successful Futures report (2015), which states that the curriculum must be relevant to a school's children and the context in which it operates, and that assessment practices must be relevant to and support the curriculum.

Phonics and reading tests

Each pupil's phonics and reading abilities are assessed at the beginning of the autumn terms and the end of both the spring and summer terms to monitor progress. The phonics test is taken from phonics sounds within the POPAT scheme and the WRaPS reading assessment is used to assess reading abilities. Results of both tests are recorded at each data point at the end of term. The results are analysed to provide further interventions to support pupil progress if necessary.

Oxford Reading Tree

Pupils using the Oxford Reading Tree have their progress tracked and attainment recorded at each data point at the end of term. The Assess and Progress Toolkit is available for teachers to use if they wish.

Self-evaluation

The school uses formative assessment (assessment for learning) to help children understand what the successful elements of their learning were so that they may be motivated to repeat them. Formative assessment helps a learner to improve in their work. Many of our children will struggle to develop meta cognition relating to their work. As such, although some practices do not necessarily involve a child reflecting on their work and developing independent meta cognition around it, they still fall firmly within the bounds of what counts as assessment for learning.

Pupils' own evaluation of their progress is actively encouraged within school. For those children able to understand, a traffic light system is used. The child chooses the colour that reflects how much help they needed to complete the task in question: whereby red equates to needing a great deal of support, amber means a little support required and green represents the ability to carry out the task independently.

Teachers will use a 'two stars and a wish' approach to marking work. Where children have the capacity to understand, the teacher may plan time for the child or the class to work with their wish to improve pieces of work or use it as a target for subsequent pieces of work. Where children are unable to understand the wish, it becomes a 'next step' for the staff member supporting them in subsequent tasks. The teacher must ensure that staff members are properly briefed on what to encourage and look out for.

A self-evaluation process for children with SLD and PMLD centres around showing them examples of their work, or a picture/film of them working, soon after completion of the task. The adult will give a social reward, explaining in a way the child may understand what element of the work was positive.

Teachers celebrate the achievements of all pupils. Some classes may use sticker charts or other tokens to support the children's motivation and forward thinking. Other classes will use recall of work through presenting work done, or pictures/films of the work being done.

It is important that teachers foster a growth mindset in their classrooms and assessment practices. Good results should be linked to the concepts of hard work, trying again and not being upset by mistakes or failures along the way.

External awards

During their time at school pupils may have the opportunity to take swimming awards, such as the ASA Water Skills awards, and riding awards administered by the Riding for the Disabled Association.

Monitoring and moderation

The assessment coordinator works to a yearly timetable of monitoring annual targets, IEPs and assessment folders to ensure good practice and school policies are maintained. The department heads will monitor use of home school diaries in the first half of autumn term, and again late in spring term.

LNF competencies are moderated internally termly, following a rolling programme across the year. Examples of moderated work are sent to a moderation network for external moderation. A teacher represents the school so that the school is represented at these meetings. The coordinators' meeting then reviews submissions by regional schools to the moderation network, in particular re-moderating failed submissions. The coordinators feed back into their local moderation arrangements.

Annual reviews and transition reviews

Every child with a Statement of Special Educational Need must have the statement reviewed annually. Every effort is made by the school to encourage parents/legal guardians to attend the annual review meeting for their child, and all professionals known to be involved with the child are also invited, including County Inclusion services. The meeting is arranged by the assessment coordinator and administrative assistant, in consultation with the class teacher. The meeting agenda follows

97

person-centred planning principles. The teacher and parents must consider whether the child should be present to contribute their views to the discussion.

The prime purpose of the review meeting is for the child's parents/legal guardians and those directly involved with the child to review progress and agree priorities for the coming year. Changes to the statement may be generated by the review meeting. Following the meeting the teacher completes the paperwork with a summary, including the main issues discussed and the agreed outcomes and priorities. Parents/legal guardians are asked to sign the annual review form and are invited to add any written comment. The school must send a copy of the final review document to the parents/ legal guardians and the County Inclusion Department within ten working days of the review meeting. The school will keep a hard copy of the review in the child's records folder in the office, and an electronic copy will also be saved into the pupil's confidential section of the school website.

Annual reports to parents

This document is produced by class teachers in June for issue towards the end of the summer term. The format will be determined by the senior management team. It provides a summary of the work covered during the academic year, reports on the responses and progress made by the pupil in each subject area and highlights any areas for future improvement. Parents are invited to reply in writing with any comments they have on the content of the report. The school is legally required to report on pupils' progress in respect of the Literacy and Numeracy Framework, so teachers will include this in each report. Although there is yet no legal requirement to do so, they will also report on the child's progress on the Digital Competence Framework.

Interdisciplinary assessment, recording and reporting

Each member of the school interdisciplinary team is responsible for assessing a pupil's needs in relation to their own area of work. In doing so they use assessment and recording parameters agreed as part of their own professional standards and contractual arrangements. However, the strength of the provision is that such information can be readily shared with both parents and class teams working with pupils.

From time to time other professionals may be involved in developing strategies for a child. This includes but is not limited to:

* Educational psychologist
* Advisory teachers for pupils with visual and/or hearing impairments
* Learning disability nurses
* Physiotherapist
* Complex needs team
* Occupational therapists
* Speech and language therapists/technicians

These professionals all have valuable roles to play to support our children's well-being and educational attainment. They may submit reports offering advice and strategies to be used with a child. All staff are expected to work constructively with fellow professionals to enhance the children's learning and welfare. All formal liaison with fellow professionals is the responsibility of the teacher.

The school's communication coordinator is responsible for liaising with SaLT services. The department heads are responsible for keeping a record of educational psychology service involvement with our children.

Home/school diaries

Diaries are used throughout the school by staff and parents to relay messages and news about home or school experiences. As most of the pupils travel on school transport, the diaries form a particularly important link between the family and the school. School staff need to be sensitive to the fact that diaries may contain confidential information and care needs to be taken as to who has access to them. Likewise, an appropriate professional tone must be used so that parents can be confident in their communication with the school.

Home school diaries will be monitored twice a year by the department heads.

Signed: (Assessment Coordinator)   **Date:**

Signed: (Headteacher)   **Date:**

Signed: (Chair of Governors)   **Date:**

Appendix 1 Assessment file contents

Assessment File Checklist for child assessed using Connecting Steps v4

Child   **Class**

Assessor   **Date**

1. Targets	
P level data × 2	
Annual targets × 2	
IEPs × 3	
LNF tracker	
3. Records	
WRaPS and phonics	
POPAT	
End Foundation and KS2 data	
ORT record	
4. Archive	
P level data sheets	
Annual Targets	
IEPs	
Music (using SOI Framework)	
WRaPS and phonics (× 3)	
POPAT records (1 year only)	
Previously completed levels	

2. Connecting Steps	
English	
Reading	
Writing	
Expressive	
Receptive	
Speaking and listening	
Maths	
Number	
Shape, space and measure	
Using and applying	
Data	
PSHE	
Citizenship	
PSHE	
Self-help	
Computing	
PE	
Welsh 2nd language	

* All above items are expected to be maintained in the assessment folder.
* Annual targets and IEPs – one piece of evidence per target.
* Connecting Steps completed levels – three pieces of evidence per level.
* Last three WRaPS and phonics tests (i.e. one year) in archive section.
* All other evidence and previous records should be removed and discarded.

Assessment File Checklist for child assessed using Autism Progress

Child   **Class**

Assessor   **Date**

1. Targets	
P level data × 2	
Annual Targets × 2	
IEPs × 3	
LNF tracker	

2. Completed Levels	
Autism Progress	
Communication	
Social Interaction	
Flexibility of Thought	
Emotional Regulation	
Connecting Steps	
Computing	
PE	
Music (using SOI)	
Welsh 2nd language	

3. Records	
WRaPS and phonics	
POPAT	
End Foundation and KS2 data	
ORT record	

4. Archive	
P level data sheets	
Annual Targets	
IEPs	
WRaPS and phonics (× 3)	
POPAT records (1 year only)	
Previously completed levels	

- All above items are expected to be maintained in the assessment folder.
- Annual targets and IEPs – one piece of evidence per target.
- Autism Progress/Connecting Steps completed levels – three pieces of evidence per level.
- Last three WRaPS and phonics tests (i.e. one year) in archive section.
- All other evidence and previous records should be removed and discarded.

Assessment File Checklist for child assessed using Routes for Learning

Child   **Class**

Assessor   **Date**

1. Targets	
RfL tracker	
P level data × 2	
Annual Targets × 2	
IEPs × 3	
LNF tracker	
2. Completed Levels	
Routes for Learning	
RfL tracker evidenced	
Connecting Steps	
Computing	
PE	
Welsh 2nd language	

3. Records	
WRaPS and phonics	
POPAT	
End Foundation and KS2 data	
ORT record	
4. Archive	
P level data sheets	
Annual Targets	
IEPs	
WRaPS and phonics (× 3)	
POPAT records (1 year only)	
Music (using SOI Framework)	
Previously completed levels	

- All above items are expected to be maintained in the assessment folder.
- Annual targets and IEPs – one piece of evidence per target.
- Routes for Learning competencies acquired – five pieces of evidence per competency.
- Connecting Steps completed levels – three pieces of evidence per level.
- Last three WRaPS and phonics tests (i.e. one year) in archive section.
- All other evidence and previous records should be removed and discarded.

Resource 13.2 Eye Gaze policy

Date:

Therapies and training programmes at our school

At our school we promote a holistic approach to the education and support we offer every pupil attending our school. We have an extensive list of therapies and training programmes that enhance the delivery of a broad and balanced curriculum to support pupils' education throughout the school. Communication is vital. Eye Gaze is a way for students to communicate who are unable with oral language, hands or other body parts. Possible candidates for Eye Gaze are: cerebral palsy, ALS, Rett syndrome, traumatic brain injury, degenerative disorders (muscular dystrophy, mitochondrial disorders).

For many Eye Gaze users, their ability to use the system is constantly changing: changes in medical status/medication; changes in physical abilities; progressive nature of some disabilities; changes in positioning; changes in their ocular motor system; changes in communicative competence; and other other (environment, education, etc.).

Eye Gaze considerations

Speech: Does the student have any use of speech and see themselves as a verbal student? Speech rate and intelligibility?

Language (receptive and expressive/pragmatics): Socially motivated. Typically, receptive skills are higher than expressive.

Cognition: Needs to be able to understand 1–2-step directions when listening to cues. Attention span in a 5–10-minute range. Able to be redirected back to task.

Physical/motor: Positioning is key! Look at how their motor patterns affect movements and stability for access.

Environment: lighting, distractibility, glare outside versus inside.

Vision: Calibration size, glasses, muscle control, long eyelashes.

Supervision

The class teacher has overall responsibility for the supervision and general safety of all those receiving a communication session or subject specific session of Eye Gaze.

Teachers and those with parental consent are responsible for furnishing the TA with any medical or behavioural issues that may be a cause for concern.

The TA will assess the pupil's suitability to receive Eye Gaze.

If concentration concerns are raised by the TA, the class teacher will observe a session to ensure the pupil is benefiting from the experience.

Eye Gaze sessions must be provided by an adult who has received the appropriate training in delivering Eye Gaze.

Data Handling – it is essential that the TA maintains appropriate and detailed records. They must ensure they are kept confidentially and adhere to data protection legislation ensuring all records held are appropriate and stored securely.

Health and hygiene

The TA must ensure they maintain a safe environment for the pupil. The room should be warm, clean and comfortable, and be free from all potential hazards. The computer system should be treated with great care and no pupil with behavioural difficulties (capable of damaging the equipment) should be permitted to access the room that the system is kept in.

Risk assessments

A risk assessment should be carried out for each pupil referred for Eye Gaze. This will include any mobility issues that may require the use of the hoist and an individual manual handling plan will be put in place if necessary. The screening forms will provide information relating to any behaviour and/or medical conditions the pupil may have, and this information must be analysed to assess any potential risk to the pupils, TA and/or equipment. If a pupil has a medical condition that requires constant monitoring, it may be deemed necessary for an additional member of staff to accompany the pupil to ensure their individual health needs are being met.

Accident procedures

All accidents or incidents that occur whilst in the room or on the way to or from the therapy room must be immediately reported to the headteacher and guidance sought from a qualified first aider if appropriate. An accident form should be obtained from the school office and completed timeously (within 24 hours of the incident/accident.).

Other guidance

It is appreciated that while every care may be taken to promote safety, there may be occasions and situations that occur despite safety precautions being in place. For such an eventuality, further clarification and advice will be sought from the headteacher who may seek further guidance from the local authority.

A. Anderson
Signed:
Chair of governors

Resource 13.3 Hydrotherapy pool policy

Supervision

The pool instructor (or session supervisor) has overall responsibility for the supervision and general safety of all those using the pool during a session.

Teachers are responsible for advising the instructor of any medical or behavioural issues that may be a cause for concern in the pool.

Sessions must be supervised by an adult with appropriate current qualifications. All sessions must have a suitably qualified adult acting as a 'spotter' on the side of the pool. This can be the pool instructor if they are not teaching the session in the water. Other adults should take care that they do not distract this person from their overall supervisory role.

The 'spotter' must not in any circumstances leave the pool area.

No pupil or client should be allowed to enter the water unless specifically directed to do so by the instructor (or session supervisor).

The instructor (or session supervisor) must check the number of pupils before they enter the water, periodically while in the water, and again when they leave.

The number of pupils/clients spectating at the pool should be kept to a minimum. They must remain seated at the changing end of the pool.

In most circumstances all users in the water should have a staff member, parent, carer, or other authorised persons to help on a one-on-one basis.

In accordance with safety guidelines in the case of an evacuation/emergency and discretion of the lead person/parties using the pool.

The responsibility in changing and travelling to and from the pool rests with the class teacher.

The pupil/client should have been toileted before entering the pool and the pupil/client wears incontinent pads or nappy in the pool if appropriate. All used nappies and tissues should be removed from pool area and disposed of appropriately.

Powered wheelchairs *must not be driven in the pool area*. When not in use these should be left in a disengaged position in a safe designated area.

Manual wheelchairs and pushchairs should only be brought into the pool area when necessary, e.g. for emergency evacuation. Pupils/clients sitting in their wheelchairs must always be supervised whilst in the pool waiting area/changing rooms.

All hoists should be returned to the appropriate docking station at the end of the session.

All slings must be returned to the appropriate storage facility when not in use.

It is essential that anyone responsible for a session in the pool familiarise himself or herself with all lifesaving equipment and the position of the alarm switch. It is helpful if as many adults as possible who normally use the pool are also aware of the location of the alarm.

Should the alarm sound during the school day, all staff who can safely leave the pupils they are immediately supervising should proceed as quickly as possible to the pool area to help.

Health and hygiene

If a 'swimmer' has a seizure in the water, the LA recommends that the information published by the RLSS should be followed, i.e. the person should be supported in the water until the attack has terminated. However, an occasion may arise where in the judgement of the pool instructor it is safer to remove the person from the water. They have the immediate responsibility for this decision.

Adults should not wear outdoor shoes in the pool area.

'Swimmers' should not use the pool if they have open wounds or dressings. The pool should not be used during menstruation unless internal protection is being used.

All swimmers are advised to shower before entering the pool.

All persons entering the pool are requested to remove shoes or wear protective covers (provided) over their shoes.

In the event of contamination of the pool by faeces or other noxious substances, the instructor supervising the session should be notified and the contamination removed using the netting provided. If diarrhoea or vomiting occurs, then the pool must be evacuated, and the caretaker notified.

Risk assessments

A risk assessment should be carried out in respect of each group using the pool. This should specify how many adults are required for safe supervision of the group both in and out of the water. Special behaviour or medical issues related to individual pupils should be listed. In the event of the specified number of adults not being present, then the pupil/s should not use the pool.

Moving and handling

Staff and support workers should follow the recommendations made by the pupils/clients handling plans.

It is the duty of all staff to alert relevant bodies/managers or teachers of any difficulties encountered in the moving and handling of pupils/clients within the pool area.

Music

The sound system installed is operated from the pool manager's office. If you have specific music that you know your student prefers, then please see the pool manager so that she may operate the system for you. We have a large selection of music and can try out different types of music with students to find their preference. We have pool switches so that the students can activate the music, light and bubble systems for themselves.

Accident procedures

All accidents/incidents at the pool during the school day must be reported immediately to the headteacher and school nurse. The normal accident report form should be obtained from the office and completed.

Other guidance

It is appreciated that the above safety precautions will not cover every eventuality. In case of doubt or for further clarification the headteacher should be asked and will seek guidance from the LA.

School pools – safety precautions

To minimise the danger of accidents during hydrotherapy sessions, headteachers and pool instructors are asked to ensure that the following safety precautions are always observed when pupils are engaged in swimming activities.

School pools

Headteachers are asked to ensure that the following items of equipment are always available:

1. At least one long safety pole, the length of which is greater than half the width of the pool
2. An adequate supply of swimming aids
3. A well-equipped first aid box
4. A telephone must always be accessible when the pool is in use

Supervision must always be provided, and hydrotherapy alone must never be permitted.
In pools shallower that one metre, a qualified lifesaver need not be present provided a *teacher or adult trained in resuscitation is present.*
Where the depth of water is restricted to two metres or less, the diving programme must be restricted to surface dive, the plunge or racing drive.
When the pool is in use, all access doors and gates must be securely locked.
Running in the pool area is not permitted.

Pool

Emergency evacuation procedure

In the event of a *medical emergency* or *collapse*, the senior member of staff is to take charge of the situation.

Pool assistant	Poolside assistant
Protect the airway and bring the casualty to the poolside	Make others aware of the emergency using the emergency button
	If an ambulance is required, then it should be called now by the school office
	(If no response from office dial _____ for direct outside line to ambulance)
	Take the evacuation board from the wall and follow user instructions
Place casualty on board as indicated	Place board in the water and allow it to scoop up the person
Secure casualty to the board with appropriate strapping	Secure casualty to the board with appropriate strapping
Rotate the board so foot end is furthest away from pool wall at a 90° angle	Rotate the board so head end is nearest the pool
Take one step forwards so that half the board is now on the side of the pool	Take one step backwards so that half the board is now on the side of the pool
Pool and poolside assistant together	
Rotate the board so that it lies at the side of the pool Ensure there is enough space to move around the casualty Commence assessment of the casualty following appropriate first aid guidelines Wet costumes to be quickly removed and casualty/surrounding area dried paying area to the chest One staff member to be present at school entrance to direct paramedics to the hydrotherapy area *Make sure other pool users are safe*	

Note: If the person is having a seizure, then they must be supported in the pool until the seizure has finished. Once stable, remove them from the pool.

Minor emergency

A minor emergency is an incident which, if handled properly, does not result in a life-threatening situation. It would normally be dealt with by the pool attendant:

- The attendant should request backup from other members of the team or responsible person.

- Either the attendant, or a delegated responsible person, should provide any treatment. The risk assessment should not be compromised. If supervision of the remaining users cannot be continued, the pool should be cleared.
- The normal reporting procedures should be used.

Major emergency

A major emergency is when an incident occurs resulting in a serious injury or life-threatening situation.

- The attendant should request backup from other members of the team or responsible person. *The alarm should be used during school hours.*
- Support team (or responsible person) should clear the pool.
- Qualified attendant rescues and initiates first aid procedures and removes casualty from the danger area.
- Support team (or responsible person) calls for an ambulance.
- Complete accident report forms and advise the headteacher.

Reporting

- Accident reporting forms are available from the school office and should be returned completed within 24 hours of the emergency.

Water quality

- If you are unable to see the bottom of the pool, the pool should be cleared immediately, and the caretaker should be informed.
- If diarrhoea or vomiting occurs, the pool should be cleared, and the caretaker informed. Once the pool is clear, any solid matter should be removed and disposed of appropriately and the area disinfected. The pool should not be reused until the pool manager has checked safety.

Fire

- If you hear the alarm, everyone should move towards the fire exit and await further instruction. If it is out of school hours, the pool area should be vacated and then meet at the muster area in the main playground and await further instruction from the fire officer in charge. *Do not return for any reason.* Full details are on notice board in the pool.

Structural and lighting failures and emission of toxic gases

Should there be any problems the pool should be cleared, and all users vacate premises by the safest route.

Resource 13.4 Meditation and mindfulness policy

Date:

This policy explains the nature of meditation and mindfulness within the school and its contribution to the education of pupils at our school. This policy has been shared and approved by the teaching staff and school governors.

Aims

Meditation and mindfulness offer pupils the opportunity to:

- Relax and develop a sense of well-being
- Enable pupils to be in the right frame of mind to learn
- Develop patience, compassion and self-awareness

Receiving meditation and mindfulness should be a personal and pleasurable experience, which enriches the lives of the pupils and those around them.

Research

Research results suggest that school-based meditation and mindfulness programmes can improve decision-making skills and teach children with special needs to focus attention and react less impulsively through breathing exercises that will allow them to reduce anxiety.

In neurotypical children, it has been shown to improve decision-making skills and to be effective in reducing anxiety (Juliano et al. 2020).

Bangor University in North Wales have a mindfulness department. A team from the university produced a paper in 2019 on the mixed experiences of mindfulness for people with intellectual disabilities (Griffiths et al. 2019). The paper reported positive changes, such as reduced aggression and increased sociability.

Entitlement

We endorse the aims of the government to provide a broad and balanced curriculum and deliver meditation and mindfulness to enable pupils to access the curriculum.

Planning

Teachers at our school match educational targets, where possible from the P levels using B Squared and from Routes for Learning (RfL). They share and discuss those targets with the parents. Teachers set different targets to meet the specific needs of individual pupils.

Equal opportunities

Meditation and mindfulness are delivered to pupils regardless of gender, culture or ability. Boys and girls have equal access to meditation and mindfulness.

Resources

Meditation and mindfulness can be delivered during other therapeutic activities such as yoga, Sherbourne dance, Tacpac, reflexology, sound bath, Qui-Gong or during an art therapy session. It can also be delivered in a daily meditation, silent or guided, throughout the week by the class teacher or a designated teaching assistant (TA). This can be done during daily activities such as eating, working and playing, and is a useful way to develop patience, compassion and self-awareness. As students' progress in their mindfulness, they can be given daily meditations to reflect on. Students would reflect on an experience and would then discuss it afterwards. This would only be for a very short time to start with, and in a designated room at our school.

Assessment, recording and reporting of pupil progress

Evaluation of learning outcomes comes from individual B Squared planning and this evaluation is used to inform future planning. The teacher records the progress made by pupils towards their targets after each session and records any evidence that the therapy has supported the well-being of the pupil. This recording sheet is copied and placed in an individual's class file. The information held in the class file provides the class teacher with the evidence to write end of session reports home to inform parents of the progress made by their child and to write reports for each pupil's annual review. An evaluation sheet is completed by the class teacher to show the impact of meditation and mindfulness on the pupil's learning and/or health.

Monitoring and evaluation of meditation and mindfulness

The therapies consultant carries out detailed monitoring and evaluation of therapies that may include meditation and mindfulness. As part of the process the consultant looks at all aspects of how they are delivered in school and the relationship to pupil progress. An action plan for further development is then drawn up. Monitoring and evaluation is carried out on a rolling programme every two years.

Supervision

The teacher has overall responsibility for the supervision and general safety of all those receiving a meditation and mindfulness session.

Those with parental consent are responsible for furnishing the teacher with any medical or behavioural issues that may be a cause for concern.

Meditation and mindfulness will *not* be administered to any pupil without parental consent.

Data handling

It is essential that the teacher maintains appropriate and detailed records. They must ensure they are kept confidentially and adhere to data protection legislation ensuring all records held are appropriate and stored securely.

Health and hygiene

The teacher must ensure they maintain a safe environment for their students. The room should be warm, clean, comfortable and be free from all potential hazards.

Risk assessments

A risk assessment should be carried out in respect of each pupil referred for meditation and mindfulness. This will provide information relating to any behaviour and/or medical conditions the pupil may have, and this information must be analysed to assess any potential risk to the pupils and/or teacher. If a pupil has a medical condition that requires constant monitoring it may be deemed necessary for an additional member of staff to accompany the pupil to ensure their individual health needs are being met.

Accident procedures

All accidents or incidents that occur whilst in the room or on the way to or from the room must be immediately reported to the headteacher and guidance sought from a qualified first aider, if appropriate. An accident form should be obtained from the school office and completed time-ously (within 24 hours of the incident/accident).

Other guidance

It is appreciated that while every care may be taken to promote safety, there may be occasions and situations that occur despite safety precautions being in place. For such an eventuality, further clarification and advice will be sought from the headteacher who may seek further guidance from the local authority.

As a rights respecting school we are committed to embedding the principles and values of the United Nations Convention for the Rights of the Child (UNCRC). This meditation and mindfulness policy ensures that our pupils have access to and are supported in the following articles of the convention.

Article 1	Every child under the age of 18 has all the rights in the Convention
Article 29	Education must develop every child's personality, talents and abilities to the full
Article 31	Every child has the right to relax, play and take part in a wide range of cultural and artistic activities
Article 42	Every child has the right to know their rights

Signed by: Chair of Governors

Resource 13.5 Sing and sign policy

Introduction

This policy explains the nature of sing and sign within the school and its contribution to the education of students at our school. This policy has been shared and approved by the teaching staff and school governors.

Content

What is sing and sign?

The sing and sign choir at our school was established when the school first opened in 2009. The choir is made up of staff and students in Key Stage 2 and promotes the use of Makaton signing whilst singing popular songs.

How does it work?

The sing and sign choir meet once a week to practise the songs and signs of popular songs. Songs are chosen based on the term's topic or events taking place across the school, such as Harvest or Easter. Staff and students also put forward any of their favourite songs. Staff are trained in Makaton and translate the words into the Makaton signs as they meet with the students during the weekly practice. The sing and sign choir perform in school and in the community during special events, such as Harvest, Christmas, Eisteddfod, Easter, Celebration of Awards, and the Leavers Service. The sing and sign choir also perform within the local community, such as for supermarkets and local care homes.

Supervision

The class teacher in charge and therapeutic music teacher have overall responsibility for the supervision and general safety of all those receiving a communication session of sing and sign.

The class teacher in charge and therapeutic music teacher will assess the student's suitability to take part in the sing and sign choir. If concentration concerns are raised by the class teacher in charge or the therapeutic music teacher, then the class teacher will observe a session to ensure the student is benefiting from the experience.

Sing and sign sessions must be provided by staff who have received the appropriate training in delivering sing and sign.

Health and hygiene

The class teacher in charge and therapeutic music teacher must ensure they maintain a safe environment for the students.

Risk assessments

A risk assessment should be carried out in respect of each student referred for sing and sign choir. This will include any mobility issues that may require the use of the hoist and an individual manual handling plan will be put in place if necessary. If a student has a medical condition that requires constant monitoring, it may be deemed necessary for an additional member of staff to accompany the student to ensure their individual health needs are being met.

Accident procedures

All accidents or incidents that occur whilst in the hall or on the way to or from the hall must be immediately reported to the headteacher and guidance sought from a qualified first aider if appropriate. An accident form should be obtained from the school office and completed timeously (within 24 hours of the incident/accident.).

Other guidance

It is appreciated that while every care may be taken to promote safety, there may be occasions and situations that occur despite safety precautions being in place. For such an eventuality, further clarification and advice will be sought from the headteacher who may seek further guidance from the local authority.

As a rights respecting school we are committed to embedding the principles and values of the United Nations Convention for the Rights of the Child (UNCRC). This Sing and Sign policy ensures that our students have access to and are supported in the following articles of the convention.

Article 1	Every child under the age of 18 has all the rights in the Convention
Article 29	Education must develop every child's personality, talents and abilities to the full
Article 31	Every child has the right to relax, play and take part in a wide range of cultural and artistic activities

Resource 13.6 Tacpac policy

This policy explains the nature of Tacpac within this school and its contribution to the education of students at our school. This policy has been shared and approved by the teaching staff and school governors.

Aims

The benefits of Tacpac include:

* A structured session whereby sensory communication is developed
* The use of objects of reference/signifiers and symbols, etc. to indicate Tacpac time
* Develops and builds trusting relationships for students to relax
* Supports non-verbal communication
* Develops self-awareness and sensory awareness
* Supports students with tactile needs

What is Tacpac?

Tacpac is a sensory communication resource using touch and music to help social and communication skills. Tacpac focuses on aligning sensory forces – it aligns the world of touch and the sensory world of music. Tacpac combines the sense of touch and music through social interaction. It is delivered via an interaction between two people – a giver and a receiver. The session is structured and takes place in an emotionally safe environment, clear of other sensory interferences.

> Tacpac is now a familiar sight and sound in most schools and settings where there is a sensory curriculum. Students may be autistic, have missing chromosomes, have global developmental delay, speech and language difficulties, attention and listening difficulties making it difficult for them to focus on aural messages, or be very wary of anyone coming close, or touching. Over time, all these students benefit from Tacpac.
>
> (http://tacpac.co.uk/tacpac-for-teachers/)

Staff teams work together on the same student each week, building a relationship over time which the student learns to trust and relax into, thereby helping non-verbal or verbal communication.

Therapies and physical development

At our school we promote a holistic approach to the education and support we offer every student attending our school. We have an extensive list of therapies that enhance the delivery of a broad and balanced curriculum of health and well-being. During these sessions students can access therapeutic interventions and activities to enhance their gross and fine motor skills.

Planning

Teachers match educational targets, where possible from the P levels using B Squared. They share and discuss those targets with the person leading the therapy. The leader and teacher may also choose targets which support the well-being of the student. Teachers set different targets to meet the specific needs of individual students.

Equal opportunities

Tacpac therapy is delivered to students regardless of gender, culture or ability. Boys and girls have equal access to this therapy.

Resources

Tacpac therapy is delivered as part of our enrichment sessions. PE mats are kept in the hall cupboard and put out by the staff member leading the session. Five blue PE mats are put out and a CD player is used. A variety of different materials are used during each session decided by the Tacpac staff member leading the session.

Assessment, recording and reporting of student progress

Evaluation of learning outcomes comes from individual B Squared planning and this evaluation is used to inform future planning. The Tacpac leader records the progress made by students towards their targets after session and records any evidence that the therapy has supported the well-being of the student; this ties into assessment purposes.

An evaluation sheet is completed by the class teacher to show the impact of the therapy on the students learning and/or health which informs part of the student's annual reviews and reports.

Monitoring and evaluation of Tacpac therapy

Teachers carry out monitoring and evaluation of sessions during enrichment sessions as well as during monitoring and evaluating time. The staff members look at aspects of gross motor development, music development and the well-being of students with links to B Squared and the new curriculum.

Supervision

Staff will meet termly to discuss and monitor the progress of areas of the curriculum and therapies across the school.

Data handling

Records of sessions are inputted directly into B Squared with observations made by the teacher/staff member carrying out therapy sessions. They must ensure they are kept confidentially and adhere to data protection legislation ensuring all records held are appropriate and stored securely.

Health and hygiene

The Tacpac leader must ensure they maintain a safe environment for their students. The TACPAC room should be warm, clean and comfortable, and be free from all potential hazards.

Risk assessments

A risk assessment should be carried out in respect of each student referred for Tacpac therapy. This will include any mobility issues that may require the use of the hoist and an individual manual handling plan will be put in place if necessary. If a student has a medical condition that requires constant monitoring it may be deemed necessary for an additional member of staff to accompany the student to ensure their individual health needs are being met. A risk assessment has been completed for the use of Tacpac therapy in the multipurpose therapy room.

Accident procedures

All accidents or incidents that occur whilst receiving Tacpac or on the way to or from the Tacpac session must be immediately reported to the headteacher and guidance sought from a qualified first aider if appropriate. An accident form should be obtained from the school office and completed timeously (within 24 hours of the incident/accident).

Other guidance

It is appreciated that whilst every care may be taken to promote safety, there may be occasions and situations that occur despite safety precautions being in place. For such an eventuality, further clarification and advice will be sought from the headteacher who may seek further guidance from the local authority.

Resource 13.7 Therapeutic music policy

Introduction

This policy explains the nature of therapeutic music and its contribution to the education of students at our school. This policy has been shared and approved by the teaching staff and school governors.

Aims

Therapeutic music offers students the opportunity to:

* Develop auditory awareness
* Develop communication, social and motor skills
* Explore musical elements
* Experience a variety of musical styles and sources
* Participate in a range of music related activities
* Develop their imagination and express themselves creatively

While learning expectations should be high, music activities should primarily provide pleasurable and creative experiences through which children can further develop confidence, communicative skill, and an aesthetic awareness of music across the world and throughout time.

The methods that therapeutic music uses begin with the premise that the child has been unable (not simply unwilling) to take part in the natural give and take of early social dialogue. We can learn to tune into their social world, and gradually help them to enter ours.

Entitlement

A variety of materials and teaching methods are used to ensure all students are engaged in the learning process. A room containing all the music resources is set aside for individual sessions. Group sessions are held in classrooms. Students also access music and the wider community by workshops, visits, performances, and visitors in and outside the school. They encounter music throughout the day during transitions (please see transition policy). They encounter music in most lessons and therapies, as it is vital in the support of their communication goals.

Content

Students are encouraged to access and explore a range of music resources, experiences and technology. This curiosity is developed and enriched through directed teaching activities led by the therapeutic music specialist.

Planning

Music as a teaching aid is recognised and utilised in all learning areas. Music is used in a variety of other curriculum areas to support learning and as a recognised aid of motivation for students.

The medium-term plans for a thematic approach to teaching and music is included in the topics, providing students with a broad and balanced curriculum, which in turn develops thinking, communication, and number and ICT skills. Teachers work closely with the therapist in music and the student's parents to ensure that the musical talents, needs and development are met for all students.

Teachers use their professional judgement and support other teachers when making decisions about transitional music to select the most appropriate for all students.

Opportunities for experiencing live music and performances are incorporated whenever possible, either at whole school performances or within departments. Students perform regularly during our Christmas, Easter and summer activities in school, as well as in supermarkets and churches found in our local community. Students are given opportunities to perform for others, either individually or as part of the group. In addition to this, students are given the opportunity to learn how to play specific musical instruments, i.e. (using keyboards, drums, etc.) in our new music club, which is run on Friday afternoons by our therapist in music.

Equal opportunities

Music is delivered to all students regardless of gender, culture or ability. Boys and girls have equal access to activities. Some students will require on-on-one therapeutic music support, and some will require group work. A therapist is employed full time to ensure that all students' music needs are met.

Within music all students are encouraged to respond to a variety of music from other cultures, the aesthetic value of music is recognised by staff, and students also have opportunities to explore this further in most other subjects and during transitions. Students regularly contribute through music to celebrations, assemblies and church services.

Special needs

All teachers must make themselves aware of any relevant medical problem or learning difficulty, which may affect a student's ability to learn. The SOWs for the subject gives suggestions for possible methods of delivery. These can be adapted to suit students by referring to the PMLD and Alternative Curriculum materials.

Within the music resources there is a selection available that have been specifically purchased to support access by PMLD students. Further adaptations ensuring access for students with sensory and/or physical impairment can be discussed and arranged with the music specialist when required.

ICT

Students use a variety of computer programs in music, as well as items such as electric keyboards, microphones and amplifiers, and iPads, Skoog, Soundbeam, etc.

Student work may be recorded using a range of audio-visual methods.

Resources

There is a wide and varied selection of resources to support students based in the music and resource room.

These can be *roughly* categorised into four areas:

1. Instruments and sound makers
2. Pre-recorded music for accompanying singing, listening and movement activities
3. Song books, resource/idea books, visual aids
4. ICT equipment and software

Music programs are also available on the interactive SMART board in classrooms. Music support is available to all staff from the therapeutic music specialist.

Assessment, recording and reporting of student progress

Please see ARR policy. Progress in music is included in the end of year report to parents, and is specific to individual participation, as well as informing on group experiences. Brief comments related to musical ability are included in the annual review reports for all students.

Monitoring and evaluation of music

The therapist in music carries out detailed monitoring and evaluation of music. As part of this process the therapist looks at all aspects of how music is delivered in school and its relationship to student progress. An action plan for further development is then drawn up. Monitoring and evaluation is carried out on a rolling programme every two years.

Health and safety

Within music staff need to be aware that many instruments are potential hazards if misused, and when working in a practical activity students should be taught how to handle apparatus appropriately. Risk assessments are always drawn up.

Possible safety issues include:

* Appropriate use of electrical equipment
* An awareness of potential choking hazards, e.g. beater heads and maraca contents
* Inappropriate use of small instruments/beaters as missiles or weapons

Review

This policy will be reviewed in the light of any changes in curriculum guidelines.

Resource 13.8 Transitional music policy

Rationale

At our school we feel it is important to create a whole school approach, of which staff, children, parents, governors and other agencies have a clear understanding. This policy is a formal statement of intent for times of transition throughout the school day.

Aim

Transitions can be a challenging time for our students, and this can lead to stress and even a 'meltdown'. This can inhibit learning.

We want our students to experience smooth, educational and emotional transitions from one place to the next and at specific agreed times during the day. This should ensure that students make the best all-round progress and promote continuity of teaching and learning. It should prevent and alleviate stress.

Equal opportunities, inclusion

The students and parents are actively involved in the process and their perceptions about transition are explored and valued. There are clear guidelines.

Principles that underpin the policy

All music/sound/songs are agreed by all staff and approved by senior management teachers, and support staff meet regularly to discuss transition times; it is an item at the weekly department meeting.

No changes are made without a whole staff meeting and approved by senior management.

There is a professional regard for information on students' ability to respond from the previous class.

Students' emotional welfare, well-being and involvement should be assessed.

Parents and carers need to be informed about the music/sound/songs used so that they may replicate them if appropriate.

The importance of transition as part of a student's learning during the day should not be overlooked.

Daily transitions should not be left to chance.

Relevant medical information is always considered.

The right amount of time is given to these important learning points of the day and they are not rushed.

123

A booklet of transition songs/sounds/music is produced for reference.

Signed: (Headteacher)   **Date:**

Signed: (Chair of Governors)   **Date:**

Resource 13.9 Vibro-acoustic therapy policy

Date:

This policy explains the nature of vibro-acoustic therapy within the school and its contribution to the education of pupils at our school. This policy has been shared and approved by the teaching staff and school governors.

Aims

Vibro-acoustic therapy offers pupils the opportunity to:

* Relax and develop a sense of well-being
* Be in the right frame of mind to learn
* Alleviate pain and discomfort

Receiving vibro-acoustic therapy should be a personal and pleasurable experience, which enriches the lives of the pupils and those around them.

Research

Research results (Lundqvist et al. 2009) indicated that self-injurious behaviours in persons with autism significantly decreased as a direct result of vibro-acoustic therapy, according to the behavioural rating instrument (completed by the person's assistant) and observational analysis.

Furthermore, assistant rating scales revealed that the participants increased in their 'sense of security' over the sessions. The authors conclude that vibro-acoustical music 'would be of benefit in the everyday life of individuals with challenging behaviours'.

Entitlement

We endorse the aims of the government to provide a broad and balanced curriculum and deliver vibro-acoustic therapy to enable pupils to access the curriculum.

Planning

Teachers at our school match educational targets, where possible from the P levels using B Squared and from Routes for Learning (RfL). They share and discuss those targets with the practitioner. The practitioner and the teacher may also choose targets which support the well-being of the pupil. Teachers set different targets to meet the specific needs of individual pupils.

Equal opportunities

Vibro-acoustic therapy is delivered to pupils regardless of gender, culture or ability. Boys and girls have equal access to this therapy.

Resources

Vibro-acoustic therapy is delivered in a designated room at our school. A vibro-acoustic bed is used to deliver this therapy and specialist music is played through the bed to provide the acoustic waves.

As the vibro-acoustic room is extremely popular and in constant use, we also have two vibro-acoustic therapy systems (music inbuilt) which are portable and can be used independently by trained assistants in classes.

Assessment, recording and reporting of pupil progress

Evaluation of learning outcomes comes from individual B Squared planning and this evaluation is used to inform future planning. The practitioner records the progress made by pupils towards their targets after each session and records any evidence that the therapy has supported the well-being of the pupil. This recording sheet is copied and placed in an individual vibro-acoustic class file. The information held in the class file provides the class teacher with the evidence to write end of session reports home to inform parents of the progress made by their child and to write reports for each pupil's annual review. An evaluation sheet is completed by the class teacher to show the impact of the therapy on the pupil's learning and/or health.

Monitoring and evaluation of vibro-acoustic therapy

The therapies consultant carries out detailed monitoring and evaluation of vibro-acoustic therapy. As part of the process the consultant looks at all aspects of how this therapy is delivered in school and its relationship to pupil progress. An action plan for further development is then drawn up. Monitoring and evaluation is carried out on a rolling programme every two years.

Supervision

The practitioner has overall responsibility for the supervision and general safety of all those receiving a vibro-acoustic therapy session.

Teachers and those with parental consent are responsible for furnishing the practitioner with any medical or behavioural issues that may be a cause for concern.

Vibro-acoustic therapy will *not* be administered to any pupil without written parental consent and the completion of a medical screening form. The practitioner will evaluate every form to assess the pupil's suitability to receive vibro-acoustic therapy. If medical concerns are raised, or any contra indications to receiving vibro-acoustic therapy are noted, oral non-objection must be sought from the pupil's general practitioner before sessions can begin.

If the practitioner has any concerns regarding potential contra indications to providing vibro-acoustic therapy, they reserve the right to refuse to treat the pupil.

Data handling

It is essential that the practitioner maintains appropriate and detailed records. They must ensure they are kept confidentially and adhere to data protection legislation, ensuring all records held are appropriate and stored securely.

Health and hygiene

The practitioner must ensure they maintain a safe environment for their clients. The treatment room should be warm, clean and comfortable, and be free from all potential hazards. The treatment bed should be covered to prevent cross contamination between pupils and any used towels washed daily using a high temperature wash. The waterbed and the therapy systems should be cleaned with a reputable surface cleaner after each session.

Risk assessments

A risk assessment should be carried out in respect of each pupil referred for vibro-acoustic therapy. This will include any mobility issues that may require the use of the hoist and an individual manual handling plan will be put in place if necessary. The screening forms will provide information relating to any behaviour and/or medical conditions the pupil may have, and this information must be analysed to assess any potential risk to the pupils and/or practitioner. If a pupil has a medical condition that requires constant monitoring, it may be deemed necessary for an additional member of staff to accompany the pupil to ensure their individual health needs are being met.

Accident procedures

All accidents or incidents that occur whilst in the therapy room or on the way to or from the therapy room must be immediately reported to the headteacher and guidance sought from a qualified first aider, if appropriate. An accident form should be obtained from the school office and completed timeously (within 24 hours of the incident/accident).

Other guidance

It is appreciated that whilst every care may be taken to promote safety, there may be occasions and situations that occur despite safety precautions being in place. For such an eventuality, further clarification and advice will be sought from the headteacher who may seek further guidance from the local authority.

As a rights respecting school we are committed to embedding the principles and values of the United Nations Convention for the Rights of the Child (UNCRC). This vibro-acoustic therapy policy ensures that our pupils have access to and are supported in the following articles of the convention.

Article 1	Every child under the age of 18 has all the rights in the Convention
Article 29	Education must develop every child's personality, talents and abilities to the full
Article 31	Every child has the right to relax, play and take part in a wide range of cultural and artistic activities
Article 42	Every child has the right to know their rights

Resource 13.10 Vibro-acoustic therapy impact report for governors – autumn term

Julie F – therapy assistant

Vibro-acoustic therapy uses sound to produce vibrations that are applied directly to the body. During the therapy pupils lie on a waterbed which is embedded with speakers. Preparation for each session involves making the room comfortable and free from interruptions with the use of support, i.e. pillows or wedges to support children/adults with physical disabilities. Specific pain management and relaxation CDs are used, with the volume kept low throughout the session so that the pupil feels the vibration rather than hears it.

During the six months that we have provided this therapy we have seen success with children and adults. There are a variety of impacts seen as a direct result of vibro-acoustic therapy around communication.

I have worked on educational targets to support communication with targets being attained. Example targets include:

- Carries two-way conversation with adult
- Asking for help
- Requesting specific music and/or session to finish.

The therapy has significantly boosted confidence, enabling pupils to converse with myself in different surroundings and build on relationships with peers.

Children/adults with physical needs gain enormously from vibro-acoustic therapy:

- Bodies visibly release tension during sessions.
- Joints, muscles show ease of movement, uncurling of fists/fingers. This has been proved when replacing clothing, splints and shoes after a session.
- Further reports have been received from adult carers that their clients become motivated for the day; and it helps with sleep patterns.
- General well-being is lifted.
- Medically it has helped children and adults with bowel problems as the low frequency tones reach organs, creating internal massage.

As the session ends the volume should be reduced slowly. During the therapy, the user may drift into a deep state of relaxation. Waking from this can be disorientating for the child/adult. Reassurance may be required to help them adjust to surroundings. I have found some children need to stretch and move around before sitting up. Overall, the therapy has had a huge impact on the children/adults using the therapy and the person delivering it.

Resource 13.11 Free music resources and support

In previous chapters I have provided links to free music support. As technology continues to improve, so will the free music. Here are some things that are available now, but I know they will continue to be supplemented, so you may wish to google the heading to find even more.

Currently the charity Oxfam provides free music lesson plans focusing on music from different parts of the world (www.oxfam.org.uk/education/resources/global-music-lessons-for-ages-7–11).

Sing Up at Home, developed during the pandemic of 2020, was made to encourage students to sing whether at home or at school. Teachers were encouraged to share the link to the school website. They have topic-related songs, and activities included songs for virtual choirs and BSL and Makaton signing videos. To find out more, go to www.singup.org.

Friday Afternoons is a site that provides singing projects for teachers and choirs. It is a free resource. To find out more, go to www.fridayafternoonsmusic.co.uk.

Portsmouth Music Hub is a free resource toolkit for schools who want to sing. They have a selection of songs to suit all abilities and occasions. Go to www.portsmouthmusichub.org.

The British Dyslexia Association (BDA) website has a section which is devoted to dyslexia and music. It also offers support in music to students with dyspraxia. Go to www.bdadyslexia.org.uk.

Melody is an organisation that promotes instrumental teaching for those with learning difficulties. To find out more, go to www.melodymusic.org.uk.

On the CBeebies channel of the BBC is a site called TenPieces. It encourages students to enjoy and take part in classical music. Each of the ten pieces of music has free resources including videos and lesson plans that can be adapted. To find out more, go to www.bbc.co.uk.

The BBC also offer BBC Teach Bring the Noise, which caters for SEND students. The site offers interactive and inclusive activities for use in school or at home.

The English Folk Dance and Song Society has specific songs for children with SEN. For instance, 'A Country Life' has Makaton lyrics to download (as well as ordinary lyrics), audio tracks to listen to and lesson plans and a host of supportive material all for free. To find out more, go to www.media.efdss.org/resourcebank.

If you have a music room that you wish to decorate with free posters on music, then go to www.nstgroup.co.uk.

If you want free access to 100 pieces of classical music, then the exam board of the Royal School of Music (ABRSM) has set up a free website for that. You will need to log in, but teachers and students get access to them. To find out more, go to www.gb.abrsm.org>classical100primary.

If you want to help students learn a musical instrument, there are many to choose from to suit their needs; we have looked at some in the chapter on technology. Apart from keyboard playing, which has proved popular with many of the students I have encountered, the ocarina is also popular, and although not free it is relatively inexpensive. It does require fine motor skills but is much easier to play than a recorder. To find out more, go to www.ocarina.co.uk.

If you want to find a regularly updated site for a list of free music resources and support, go to www.musicmark.org.uk.

Resource 13.12 Therapeutic music report for parents

_____Term

The aim of the use of therapies at our school is to enable pupils to be in the right frame of mind to learn.

Pupil:_____Class:_____

B Squared/Routes for Learning targets that we have been working on/achieved.

These are targets that have been set by the class teacher. They work alongside the IEP's set for the term.

Therapeutic targets

These are targets that have been set by me as the therapist to work alongside teacher-recommended targets.

Report recommendations (highlighted below)

Has come to the end of a six-week block of therapeutic music sessions.

Will be reassessed for further sessions in _____ term.

Will continue with Therapeutic music sessions.

Signed: _____ therapist

Table 13.1 Soundbeam targets

Name: **Term:**

Class: **Teacher:**

Number

➢ To ask for 'more' using PECS

Computing

➢ Operates control device (switch/paddle) in response to visual prompt (P4)

➢ To develop an understanding of cause and effect (relates action to sound)

Figure 13.1 Soundbeam targets

Individual Session Recording

Name: **Term:**   **Class:**

Teacher: **Therapist:**

Target – Picture Evidence: BSquared P level:	Target – Comments –
Comments –	Comments –
Comments –	Comments –

Evaluation	Any Suggestions

Table 13.2 POPAT AIT research data

POPAT progress using AIT 2015–2016 POPAT follows the normal course of language development stimulating speech and listening			
Students are assessed in April every year on their POPAT progress. Students below were nor making progress with POPAT in April 2015. Only when these are mastered does it teach a written system. Listening is a big part of the programme.			
Pupil:	**Date AIT received**	**Autumn 2015**	**Spring 2016**
RD	April 2015	Game 1a/1b Listen and choose	Game 1a/1b Listen and choose
SH	June 2015	Game 1a/1b Listen and choose	Game 4 Listen and choose
EG	June 2015	Game 5 Foundation	Transition 2 Listen and choose
EB	September 2015	Game 4 Listen and choose	Transition 2 Listen and choose
RC	October 2015	Game 2 Foundation	Game 3 Foundation
JM	October 2015	Game 1a/1b Listen and choose	Game 3 Listen and choose
CS	November 2015	Game 2 Listen and choose	Game 4 Listen and choose
JS	November 2015	Transition 1 Listen and choose	Transition 1 Listen and choose

Does AIT improve students listening skills?

Progress shown has been outstanding for most students selected. They were not given any additional POPAT support. RD, who did not make any progress, has had some big changes in his life which have affected his approach to learning and participation in learning. JS also did not make any progress. Both boys will now be offered Irlen lens therapy this term, and if it has no effect, we will decide as to whether POPAT is a suitable phonics programme for both.

Table 13.3 Risk assessments

Directorate		Activity (Brief description)	Therapeutic music room		
Service	Education	**People at risk**	Pupils and staff		
Location		**Date**		**Review date**	ongoing
Assessor		**Issue number**	1		
Item No	**Hazard (include defects)**	**Risk rating (without controls) High/Medium/Low**	**Existing control measures**		**Risk rating (with existing controls) High/Medium/Low**
	General Storage Falling instruments/ equipment Not secured, poorly installed. Sited too high/overloaded	Medium	Storage unit professionally installed and fixings in place. Storage to be organised. Restricted access to pupils. Controlled limits of items stored.		Low
	Cleanliness and tidiness Tripping Mouthing of instruments/ equipment by student	Medium	Rubbish is regularly removed. Equipment tided away after activity has finished. Clean equipment after every session.		Low
	Lone working Working in music room alone/in an isolated location Accident, injury, delayed assistance in emergency	Medium	Only agreed tasks to be undertaken. Reduced time spent working alone so far is reasonably practicable. Clear boundaries set. Staff member allowed use of phone in case of emergency. Room is nearby _____ classroom who is onsite in the event of summoning assistance.		Low

(Continued)

(Continued)

Injury	High	Staff support throughout activities. Carefully selected instruments and equipment Staff trained in basic first aid. Room is nearby to _____ classroom who is onsite in the event of summoning assistance. Risk assessments of individual pupils carried out before beginning music if this is a known behaviour by pupil.	Low
Behavioural issues	Medium	Pupils IBP in individual folder and followed by staff. Staff aware of pupil's IBP. Clear boundaries set at start. Staff trained in positive behaviour strategies and de-escalation techniques. Adequate staffing required if necessary. Risk assessments of individual pupils carried out before beginning therapeutic music. Room is nearby to _____ classroom who is onsite in the event of summoning assistance.	Low
Medical issues	High	Pupils care plans in place and followed by staff. Staff aware of pupil's medical needs and rescue meds taken to room. Staff trained in medical needs. Adequate staffing required if necessary. Risk assessments of individual pupils carried out before beginning therapy if necessary. Room is near _____ classroom who is onsite in the event of summoning assistance.	Low

Further action required to reduce risks to acceptable level

			low
Consideration given to staff at increased risk, e.g. new or expectant mothers, inexperienced staff, etc. and lone working activities avoided where practicable.	medium		low
Safeguarding		Therapist to follow safeguarding procedures of school and to have attended safeguarding training	
Risk assessments of individual pupils' medical and/or behavioural needs carried out before beginning therapy if necessary			
Ultimate risk	*High*	*Ultimate existing risk*	*Low*

Item no.	Further action necessary to control risk	Action by	Date completed	Residual risk (with further controls) High/Medium/Low

Assessor(s) signature(s)	Manager's name	Manager's signature

Other relevant risk assessments:

Table 13.4 Music, sound and vibrations skills ladder

AoLE areas: Expressive and therapeutic arts

Subject	Strand	P4	P5	P6
Music	Controlling sounds –performing skills	• Shows some care when using instruments	• Identifies where equipment goes	• Matches pictures of instruments
		• Explores a range of instruments in staff-led group activity	• Shares the same central equipment source	• Communicates what they are going to do, e.g. hit/scrape
		• Helps to hand out objects to a group when asked	• Repeats an action that created laughter	• Observes an adult playing an instrument
		• Joins in rhymes or jingles	• Plays an instrument in a group	• Tries to play an unfamiliar instrument
		• Plays simple musical instruments	• Shows an awareness of the purpose of equipment	• Shows interest in unfamiliar instrument
		• Makes a variety of vocal sounds	• Uses equipment appropriately	• Puts equipment in box provided
		• Deliberately makes sounds with body	• Takes part in a performance with others	• Helps an adult collect equipment from group, e.g. books/musical instruments
		• Claps hands with others	• Starts and stops playing in response to signal from conductor	• Tries to use knowledge of familiar equipment when trying new equipment

(Continued)

	• Activates a piece of music in pool/therapy room • Matches a picture to transitional music destination • Starts and stops a sound on classroom instruments	• Searches out specific instrument: drum, triangle, shake, tambourine and maracas	• Uses body to create different sounds • Maintains silence • Points to an instrument that can be shaken/hit
Creating and developing musical ideas – composing skills	• Repeats an action to obtain a similar effect • Points to favourite instrument • Can remain focused on own activity • Can be drawn into an activity • Copies an action made on an instrument, demonstrating similar physical movements • Copies/imitates a sound of an instrument • Communicates with peers enthusiastically	• Works alongside a peer without support from a member of staff • Chooses to work or play alongside another pupil • Works with two others with assistance • Repeats activity to refine skill • Makes a sound, gesture or movement and expects a specific reaction • Selects an instrument by function, e.g. striking/shaking to make a sound • Copies simple rhythm	• Imitates others to create a sound either on an instrument or vocally • Describes a simple sequence of actions • Explores sound using a simple computer program • Feels and simply describes vibrations on a drum or resonance board • Takes turns to make sounds with their instruments • Follows picture symbols to make sounds which are: high, low, loud and quiet

139

(Continued)

Responding and reviewing – appraising skills		
• Seeks sound source • Listen to meditation/AIT/neurofeedback music for 1 minute • Demonstrates anticipation when specific equipment is distributed • Moves body to music • Moves rhythmically to music • Makes/activatse noises in response to a picture, e.g. car, cat, etc. • Makes vocal or physical sounds/activates sounds in response to music • Communicates what they are doing • Responds when an error occurs in a familiar song/rhyme	• Communicates simply about a piece of music • Shows reaction to meditation activity • Joins in adult-led action rhymes • Remains focused on staff-led meditation music/AIT/neurofeedback for 5 minutes • Looks for a response to shouting • Moves to music • Stops and starts when the music begins and finishes • Plays 'statues', stopping as the music stops • Answers simple questions about music heard • Responds to changes in sound or music with body movements • Communicates simply what was successful about their performance	• Communicates what they are doing and gives a reason, using words, signs or symbols • Responds appropriately to familiar equipment used by therapist • Responds appropriately to the music of others • Claps hands to show appreciation • Experiments with moving to music in different ways • Movement terms – with object or person: stop, start, up, down, high, low, fast and slow. • Responds appropriately when transition music starts • Imitates movement using simple rhythms • Uses karaoke equipment • Watches self on a clip and communicates recognition

Listening and applying knowledge and understanding	• Notices changes in sound of environment • Uses visual and audible indications that signal events, e.g. sound of table being set • Relates a range of everyday sounds to events • Correctly identifies sounds when listening to recorded sounds • Turns towards or quietens when hearing a peer cry • Remains on task for 2/3 minutes	• Listens with headphones • Listens to an audiobook • Listens to self on recording • Follows two simple directions • Echo teacher in producing animal sounds • Identifies the sound source when an object is out of view • Tries to echo a short melody with their voice • Imitates sounds which are: loud, quiet, quick and slow • Imitates specific sound made on an instrument • Listens to performance/ presentation of others	• Listens to adults when offering choice • Listens to a recording of themselves and friends with interest • Recognises speech of familiar people on audio • Recalls some sound sources • Listens to a peer making a sound • Identifies equipment that uses electricity, e.g. iPad/keyboards • Uses simple criteria to describe music: happy, sad, slow and fast • Listens for and tries to identify sounds in the classroom • Listens for and tries to identify sounds in the school grounds

Subject	Strand	P7	P8	NC1
Music	**Controlling sounds through singing and playing – performing skills**	• Expresses their feelings through creative work	• Shows pride in their group's achievements	• Completes call and response melodies
		• Treats equipment with care	• Stays on task in group situation with assistance	• Sings/signs action songs
		• Accepts they may have to wait to use specific equipment	• Cooperates to achieve a simple task	• Sings/signs songs with and without an accompaniment
		• Shares equipment	• Uses puppets, giving them a voice	• Mouths/chants/creates noise in time with an accompaniment
		• Interacts while sharing equipment	• Contributes to making sounds	• Able to speak/sign/choose rhymes
		• Works in pairs	• Participates by clapping along to music	• Explores and communicates the different sounds from one instrument
		• Works in small groups	• Selects an instrument to play	• Suggests which instrument would make a certain sound
		• Takes turns	• Works in a group (lead by adult) to rehearse	• Holds simple instruments correctly
		• Explores a range of musical instruments, demonstrating what they have found out	• Decides who will play when	• Follows the lead to clap or walk to pulse
		• Plays an instrument at same time as another	• Follows a simple graphic score	• Makes sound effects for stories/poems

	• Chooses two people to join an activity • Picks the instrument which corresponds to symbols on a graphic score • Knows when to begin/stop playing or singing in echo activity	• Plays from a graphic score • Prompts a member of their group to play • Performs a solo • Performs in a group • Likes to try new instruments • Makes different sounds from one instrument • Tries different methods of gaining new sounds from instruments	• Rehearses with others in small group • Watches and follows the conductor to know when to: start/stop, get louder/quieter, speed up/slow down • Sings with an awareness of other performers
Creating and developing musical ideas – composing skills	• Communicates what they are going to do, giving a reason • Observes changes in sound • Records sounds around school • Plays notes using comparatives: longer, quieter, louder and quieter	• Creates sounds to accompany a story, picture, feeling, etc. • Communicates which instrument should play next • Repeats action to refine movement	• Creates rhythmic pattern to a given pulse • Creates a rhythmic sequence which changes tempo • Creates a pattern which shows a contrast in dynamics • Represents high and low sounds visually using simple patterns or picture symbols

(Continued)

(Continued)

• Chooses specific pictures to symbolise high or low notes • Orders symbols from left to right • Chooses symbols in a computer program to create sound patterns • Whilst playing a rhythm, can play louder, quieter, faster and slower • Points to symbols on a graphic score whilst the music is being played • Improvises a simple rhythm • Chooses an instrument which creates a specified sound • Repeats a rhythmic pattern	• Explores computer software to create new sound patterns • Creates sound effects • Imitates sound played on the same instrument which could be quiet/loud, long/short • Uses body signs to show a high/low sound • Composes music with symbols to represent long/short sounds • Composes music with symbols to represent high/low notes • Composes music with symbols to represent loud/quiet notes • Chooses an instrument to do a specific job	• Creates a short musical sequence that combines long and short sounds • Creates a musical sequence which has a beginning and an end • Includes repetition in their compositions, e.g. in rhythms or melodies • Acts as conductor to begin/end their music • Makes contribution in whole class/group compositions • Changes sounds on an electronic keyboard

Responding and reviewing – appraising skills		
• With support, answers questions about an activity	• Expresses their feelings through movement	• Dance movements begin to show awareness of pulse
• Responds to other people's ideas	• Makes a collection of instruments that satisfy a condition, e.g. can be shaken	• Responds to music using body percussion
• Moves using simple rhythms	• Answers questions about what they are doing	• Makes up simple dance patterns
• Explores basic body actions in Sherbourne dance	• Changes movements spontaneously with music	• Responds to mood changes when dancing
• Recognises self on audio	• Stops Sherbourne dance when music stops	• Suggests reasons why they like a certain piece or style of music
• Shows appreciation of a performance, e.g. clapping	• Creates a short dance sequence using a variety of actions	• Draws a shape which describes a sound
• Demonstrates appropriate audience behaviour, e.g. listening quietly	• Watches and discusses movement	• Uses key word when describing what they did
• Communicates about how the music makes them feel	• Discusses their work using appropriate vocabulary	• Comments on differences in others' work
• Records their activity and results, e.g. selects the correct picture in a sequence		• Listens to a recording of their music and says which parts worked best
• Is aware of volume		• Changes their idea if it does not work

(Continued)

(Continued)

Listening and applying knowledge and understanding	• Correctly uses comparative terms: high/low, top/bottom, stop/start, on/off, fast/slow, big/small • Identifies sounds on audio • Plays sound lotto • Listens to rhymes carefully • Understands that music is part of celebrations and daily life • Identifies the musicians in school	• Makes simple musical instrument • Describes the notes heard using the words 'high' and 'low' accurately • Describes a sequence of three notes • Tries to give a reason for their opinion • Becomes aware of the use of an external microphone	• Communicates how the music made them feel • Shows enjoyment when listening to songs • Identifies personal preferences for songs • Evaluates music they have heard using simple words	• Listens for and pinpoints long and short sounds in a piece of recorded music • Listens for and pinpoints high and low sounds in a piece of music • Recognises the difference between loud and quiet sounds, and silence • Recognises rhythmic patterns by singing/playing them back • Watch a performance from a visiting musician	• Identifies simple processes they need to develop to improve their work • Identifies a new skill they have developed

• Communicates if music is fast/ slow • Listens to longer pieces of music without disruption	• Listens to a piece of music quietly • Identifies the roles of a musician in the community • Able to communicate whether a note is high/ low, quiet/loud, fast/ slow	• Pinpoints the beginning, middle and end of a song • Recalls songs or sound patterns from memory • Identifies different sound sources • Can determine between one strand or more than one strand of music

Subject	Strand	NC2
Music	**Controlling sounds through singing and playing – performing skills**	• Demonstrates awareness of pitch when following the shape of a melody whilst singing
		• Breathes at the end of a phrase when singing
		• Confidently sings songs with others
		• Listens to others whilst singing
		• Sings with the correct posture
		• Performs a rhythm to a given pulse
		• Responds to two instructions when performing music, e.g. louder and faster
		• Controls the level of dynamics when playing a tuned or untuned instrument
		• Holds and plays simple instruments correctly
		• Claps the 'rhythm' or syllables of a word or phrase
		• Decides how some orchestral instruments could be played
		• Selects an instrument for a specific sound
		• Can change the sound of an instrument
		• Performs a short piece alone and in a group with symbols as support

	• Is quiet before and at the end of a song
	• Records their music
Creating and developing musical ideas – composing skills	• Creates a sequence of sounds which have a beginning, middle and end
	• Uses symbols to plan a sequence of sounds
	• Plays or claps from their simple notation, e.g. graphical
	• Creates rhythmic patterns which includes rests
	• Creates a short vocal melodic pattern
	• Score includes dynamic instruction
	• Includes the use of silence (rests) in their composition
	• Understands that notes can be repeated when composing
	• Finds the first few notes of a well-known song, e.g. 'Three Blind Mice'
	• Makes up/retells story using tuned instruments to represent a character
	• Makes improvements to their compositions
	• Directs others in a group
Responding and reviewing – appraising skills	• Able to move to music relating to low/high stepwise/jumping sounds
	• Creates a dance movement to represent a sound from contrasting instruments

(Continued)

(Continued)

	• Uses onomatopoeic words to describe sounds
	• Moves to the pulse of the music
	• Communicates about music they like, commenting on musical elements
	• Communicates about music they have heard
	• Shows the direction of pitch with their hand
	• Brainstorms words which describe the music
	• Draws a picture which represents the sounds/music heard
	• Communicates about the words and meanings in seasonal songs
	• Evaluates a piece of music using a simple grid as a guide
	• Watches a video of their performance and discusses/signs/communicates what could be improved
Listening and applying knowledge and understanding	• Identify similar rhythmic patterns
	• Hears the difference between a male and female voice
	• Able to tap the pulse whilst listening to a recording of their music
	• Names/signs/communicates tuned and untuned classroom instruments correctly
	• Hears when music is getting higher or lower

- Understands that tempo relates to speed

- Recognises sounds which move in steps and leaps

- Classifies timbres in simple terms

- Watches and discusses (using appropriate communication tools) a performance from a visiting musician

- Identifies tempo as: fast, slow, moderate, getting slower and getting faster

- Recognises crescendo and diminuendo

- Makes a sound map of their school

- Knows movement can create sound

- *Explains that we hear sounds when they reach the ear*

Table 13.5 Vibro-acoustic therapy (VAT) screening form

Name of student	
Date of birth	
Address	
Telephone number	
Name and telephone number of emergency contact	
Primary diagnosis	
Any other relevant factors	
Weight	
Height	

Important

If you answer *yes* to any of the questions, please consult your GP to ask if they have any objection to your child using VAT and sign in the appropriate space below.

Please answer with as much detail as possible if you answer *yes* to any question.

Does the person named overleaf suffer from any of the following?

Condition	Yes	No
Recent heart attack or coronary disease		
Psychotic conditions		
Pregnancy (adults/staff member)		
Diabetes		
Epilepsy		
Head or neck injuries after an accident		
Acute states, like thrombosis or angina pectoris		
Bulge of intervertebral disc		
Active or acute inflammation		
Pacemaker		
Acute haemorrhage (this does not include menstruation)		
Hypotension/hypertension		
Arthritis		
Recent accident, head, neck injuries, fractures, sprains or injuries		
Serious acute infections (excluding normal flu)		

If you have answered *yes* to any of the questions above, please sign below to say you have obtained your GP's oral non-objection.

Signed: **Date:**

By signing this declaration, you agree to follow any protocols put in place to ensure the safety of students.

SIGNED:	(signature of applicant or on behalf of)
PRINT NAME:	
DATE:	
School use: **Received and assessed by:**	**Date:**

Table 13.6 Visual analogue scale

A visual analogue scale allows you to mark a cross in red before the therapy begins on how the student feels regarding the areas below. A parent or teacher may need to assist with this if the student is unable to communicate to the therapist.

Once treatment sessions are completed the scale may be revisited and a black cross marked where the student feels they are now (or where the parent or teacher feels they are).

General arousal

Restless ———————————————————————— Calm

Mood

Depressed ——————————————————————Happy

Relaxation

Tense ———————————————————— Relaxed

Pain

Unbearable ————————————————Painless

Quality of sleep

Bad ———————————————————— Good

Range of movement

Spastic ———————————————— Flexible

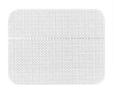

Appendix

1 E-Tran frame

An E-Tran frame is a sheet of stiff, transparent Perspex onto which symbols, letters or words can be stuck with Blu-Tack or Velcro. The student then eye-points to the symbol/letter/word to make up words or sentences that they wish to communicate. The communication partner faces the user and the frame is between them. Initially the letter or symbol will be placed in each corner. As the student becomes more skilled at eye pointing more are added to the frame. Sometimes a person may move onto use an Eye Gaze machine.

2 Niemann Pick C disease

Niemann Pick C disease is a degenerative genetic disorder. Harmful quantities of fatty substances, called lipids, accumulate in the spleen, liver, lungs, bone marrow and brain. Niemann Pick disease is divided into four types: A–C2. There is no effective treatment for type A. Gene therapies may help type B. There is currently no known cure for Niemann Pick C disease, though a drug called Miglustat has been shown to stabilise certain neurological conditions. In my experience, it is a progressive disease that worsens as the child ages. They may become wheelchair-bound as a young teenager. I have found that when depression set in for a particular teenage student (her sister had died of the same disease), music was her solace. Please go to npuk.org to find out more about the disease.

3 Cockayne syndrome

Cockayne syndrome is a rare disease which causes noticeably short stature, premature ageing (progeria), severe photosensitivity, and moderate to severe learning difficulties. It also includes failure to thrive in the new-born, very small head (microcephaly), and impaired nervous system development. Other symptoms can include hearing loss, tooth decay, vision problems and bone decay. There are three subtypes. Type 2 is the most severe and affected people do not survive past childhood. This is the subset I am most familiar with. There is no cure at present for Cockayne syndrome. Treatments may include different therapies, sometimes a gastrostomy tube placement, and medication. Sleeping is a problem and one of our students found both hydrotherapy and therapeutic music settled her at the end of the day, and she was able to sleep through the night. To find out more, go to https://cockaynesyndrome.org.

4 West syndrome

West syndrome is characterised by a specific type of seizure seen in infancy and childhood. West syndrome leads to developmental regression with each and every seizure. Seizures are scary to watch and so must be very frightening to experience. Spasms often occur in clusters of up to 100 at a time. Infants may have up to dozens of these clusters in a day. Infantile spasms tend to peter out by the age of five but are replaced by other types of seizures. There may be an underlying cause for the spasms but sometimes there is not. In my experience students with West syndrome are on a lot of antiepileptic drugs and several medications. There are different levels of West syndrome. In my experience, students have responded well to Eye Gaze and are able to play the keyboard using it. I have seen students with West syndrome leave school at 19 to live in residential care. I have supported a residential centre with setting up switches so that a young man with West syndrome could control the music he wished to hear rather than the music the carers chose for him. I have mourned the death of a beautiful young girl with West syndrome aged only ten. All of the students with West syndrome I have worked with have been wheelchair-bound. To find out more, go to www.epilepsy.org.uk.

5 Dravet syndrome

Dravet syndrome is a rare, catastrophic, lifelong form of epilepsy beginning in the first year of life. The prolonged seizure happens in the first year of life and developmental delays become evident in the second or third year. In my experience, the seizure continues and can be prolonged. There is delayed speech and in some instance no speech. Parents tell me there are sleep difficulties. Vibro-acoustic therapy can help. Students are often absent with chronic infections. We had a wonderful photo in school of a lovely little boy with Dravet syndrome laughing as he enjoyed a particular piece of music. He died aged six. For more information, go to Dravetfoundation.org.

6 Sanfilippo syndrome

Sanfilippo is a rare genetic condition also known as mucopolysaccharidosis type 111. It causes fatal brain damage. It is a type of childhood dementia and most do not reach adulthood. It is sometimes hard to diagnose and I remember a particular parent who was very persistent with her doctors, who felt her six-year-old son, Oliver, had ADHD problems. Gene testing provided the answer she really did not wish to hear, and I accompanied her on a weekend away where we got to find out more about the syndrome and how we as a school and they as parents could help.

As a young boy he would be totally unpredictable and hyperactive due to the brain damage (over time the brain cells fill up with waste that the body was unable to process). I vividly remember walking down the corridor when he, aged seven, ran from nowhere and slapped me across the face. We are taught in special schools to respond in a gentle non-threatening manner, which I did. I also recall a few weeks later when he did the same at our local Riding for the Disabled and he hit an RDA walker who hit him back. Needless to say, an investigation entailed, and she was banned from working with children. I also recall another boy with the syndrome, Russell, aged 13, whom I'd taught previously. He was wheelchair-bound, could not speak, was immobile and constantly in hospital with infections. He died aged 13. That is what the other young boy had to look forward to. Knowing that, as I did, how could you show anything but compassion? Both boys responded well to music. To find out more, go to Sanfilippo.org.au.

7 Sounds of Intent Framework

The aim of Sounds of Intent is to investigate and promote the musical development of children and young people with learning difficulties. The 'Sounds of Intent' research project was set up in 2002 jointly by the Institute of Education, Roehampton University, and the Royal National Institute of the Blind.

A framework of musical development covers the whole range of ability, from profound and multiple learning difficulties (PMLD) to those with autism, attention deficiency hyperactive disorder (ADHD), etc. The framework is freely available to anyone who wishes to use it, and works on all platforms, including touch-screen technology (such as iPads). The software enables ideas for promoting children's engagement with music to be viewed and downloaded, and for individual children to be assessed.

* The heart of the Sounds of Intent website is the framework.
* The framework is available as text or as an interactive graphic.
* There are three domains – Reactive, Proactive and Interactive.
* There are six levels which begin from the inside circle (level 1) to the outside circle (level 6).
* There are four different elements (A, B, C, D) within each level descriptor.
* A navigation tool, which is a menu box, follows you wherever you go on the website.
* There are interpretations and strategies on how to develop the activities and a selection of videos giving examples of some musical activities that relate to that domain and level.
* You can input session data, which records and translates the information you provide and then creates a graph where you can clearly see the pupil's developments and progressions.
* The website has everything required to make pupil assessments, record data and create tables and graphs to reflect the record of interactions.
* There is a video on the home page of the website called 'Sounds of Intent Young Champions' where a group of young people have created a clear guide on how to use SOI.
* Teachers, therapists, other practitioners and parents can register to assess their children online. Assessments can be made as a one-off or over a period of time. The results can be printed out as numbers or in graphical form.

* It can support pupils in highlighting their musical skills and creativity backed up with video footage.
* It makes clear comparisons with the 'P levels' for music and their limitations.
* It is a quick and reliable way to record and save session data.
* You can generate and print a table and graph based on the data entered.

You can study for a Postgraduate Certificate in Sounds of Intent through the University of Roehampton. Go to www.roehampton.ac.uk/postgraduate-courses/sounds-of-intent/.

The certificate offers students an introduction to the framework for children and young people with special educational needs and disabilities (SEND) and professional development to meet those needs.

Students are introduced to the SOI Framework and learn how to use the resources and assessment tool available through the website. The course has both theoretical and practical elements and is assessed through essays, a portfolio of work and a placement.

The resource has taken over ten years to research and develop, involving hundreds of practitioners from across the special education sector. The tool is made up of three components: an online assessment tool, a curriculum framework and downloadable resources.

The Sounds of Intent qualification will support those seeking work through music in special schools.

8 Routes for Learning (RfL) Framework

Routes for Learning was first published in 2006 and was updated in 2019. It is assessment material for learners with PMLD and SLD. It focuses on early communication, social interaction and the cognitive skills that are crucial for learning. This assessment material helps teachers to take account of a learner's preferred learning channel (e.g. auditory, visual, tactile), their way of communicating, anticipation, problem solving and social skills. It is not subject-specific. Only the SOI Framework is subject-specific. To find out more about RfL, go to hwb.gov.wales.

9 Engagement Model

The Engagement Model assessment tool is to support staff in maintained schools including special schools, academies, pupil referral units, hospital schools and MOD schools in England. They are not mandatory for non-maintained or independent schools. The model replaces P scales 1–4 and becomes statutory 2020/21. It is not subject-specific.

10 Quest for Learning Model

Go to ccea.org.uk to find out more.

11 Schumann vibrations

The Schumann frequencies are quasi-standing electromagnetic waves that exist in the space between the surface of the Earth and the ionosphere. Driven by lightning, and affected by solar flares, these primal Schumann resonance pulses are thought to calibrate us and enhance our physical and mental well-being. In1954 Schumann and Herbert König reported the fundamental frequency to be 7.83 Hz. König showed that human reaction times were significantly correlated with the intensity of the 8–10 Hz Schumann signal (Saroka et al. 2014). Research carried out by E. Jacobi at the University of Düsseldorf showed that the absence of Schumann waves creates mental and physical health problems in the human body. NASA has been greatly interested in the Schumann resonances following the first space missions with astronauts. Their research study findings indicated that cells grow faster and stronger and live longer when exposed to low frequency pulsed electromagnetic fields like the Schumann resonances (Goodwin 2003). This research was a significant contribution toward enabling humans to live and work safely in space.

12 Entrainment

In 1656 Dutch mathematician, physicist and astronomer Christian Huygens formulated the principle of entrainment. Entrainment describes a process whereby two rhythmic processes interact with each other in such a way that they adjust towards and eventually 'lock in' to a common phase and/or periodicity (Clayton et al. 2004).

13 Resonance

In 1898 Nikola Tesla published a paper 'High Frequency Oscillators for Electro-Therapeutic and other purposes' (Tesla 2014). A quote from the paper reads: 'The cell with very weak vibrations, when placed in the field of multiple vibrations, finds its own frequency and starts again to oscillate normally through the phenomenon of resonance'.

14 Sound frequency

In early 1900 Dr Albert Abrams was an expert in neurology and discovered that using sound frequency was curative (Lutz 1995).

15 Radio frequencies

In 1925 George Lakhovsky published a paper, 'Curing cancer with Ultra Radio frequencies' in *Radio News* (Lakhovsky 1925).

16 Royal Rife

In 1934 Dr Royal Raymond Rife successfully cured 16 patients of cancer by using his hand-built vibration frequency device. The American Medical Association did not support Rife and banned the use of his device to treat patients. It is speculated that a pharmaceutical conspiracy was the root cause (Lynes 1987).

17 Binaural beats

In 1973 Gerald Oster suggested that it could be possible to diagnose and address neurological problems using binaural beats, with the potential to address problems such as stress and anxiety, insomnia, memory/cognitive decline, pain relief and more. The process behind the creation of binaural beats enables us to isolate particular frequencies that have been shown to positively influence the brain in a particular way (Oster 1973).

18 Stimming

Stimming is a shortened term for self-stimulatory behaviour. Students with autism can sometimes be seen hand flapping, spinning, jumping, using a fidget toy, or asking repeated questions, or saying words or phrases. In the distant past these behaviours were frowned upon and discouraged. Nowadays fidget toys are big business and are popular everywhere. It is realised that a fidget toy can help concentration and focus the mind. A fidget toy is a little like a safety valve helping to reduce the pressure of the situation. Virtual assistants such as Alexa, Siri and Cortana can aid students who get into the spiral of continuous questioning.

19 Somatron (www.biof.com/somatron/pain_ management.asp)

Level 1 – balance: This is the most widely used breath-based stress reduction composition, and still the healing profession's defining benchmark for eliciting the Relaxation Response. It is used by hospitals, stress reduction clinics and healthcare facilities around the world.

Level 2 – serenity: This is a composition that will allow the listener to settle into the relaxation experience. Level 2 makes use of the subconscious resonances associated with the water archetype, encouraging the listener to breathe deeply and relax and let go of the tensions that prolong chronic pain.

Level 3 – tranquillity: This composition brings forward the Relaxation Response at its deepest level.

Level 4 – harmony: While equally relaxing, this composition takes a different approach. This piece should bring a high degree of pain reduction even to your most difficult of cases.

20 P levels

Otherwise known as P scales, these supplement the national curriculum by specifying performance attainment targets (P scales) and performance descriptors for pupils aged 5–16 with special educational needs (SEN) who cannot access the national curriculum. They are now no longer statutory in England, although schools continue to use them for guidance purposes. They have been used as non-statutory guidance in other countries. Below is the published guidance for music P levels.

Music performance descriptors

P1 (i) pupils encounter activities and experiences

* They may be passive or resistant.
* They may show simple reflex responses (for example, startling at sudden noises or movements).
* Any participation is fully prompted.

P1 (ii) pupils show emerging awareness of activities and experiences.

* They may have periods when they appear alert and ready to focus their attention on certain people, events, objects or parts of objects (for example, becoming still in a concert hall).
* They may give intermittent reactions (for example, sometimes becoming excited at repeated patterns of sounds).

P2 (i) pupils begin to respond consistently to familiar people, events and objects.

* They react to new activities and experiences (for example, turning towards unfamiliar sounds).
* They begin to show interest in people, events and objects (for example, looking for the source of music).
* They accept and engage in coactive exploration (for example, being encouraged to stroke the strings of a guitar).

P2 (ii) pupils begin to be proactive in their interactions.

* They communicate consistent preferences and affective responses (for example, relaxing during certain pieces of music but not others).
* They recognise familiar people, events and objects (for example, a favourite song).
* They perform actions, often by trial and improvement, and they remember learned responses over short periods of time (for example, repeatedly pressing the keys of an electronic keyboard instrument).
* They cooperate with shared exploration and supported participation (for example, holding an ocean drum).

P3 (i) pupils begin to communicate intentionally.

* They seek attention through eye contact, gesture or action.
* They request events or activities (for example, leading an adult to the CD player).
* They participate in shared activities with less support.
* They sustain concentration for short periods.
* They explore materials in increasingly complex ways (for example, tapping piano keys gently and with more vigour).
* They observe the results of their own actions with interest (for example, listening intently when moving across and through a sound beam).
* They remember learned responses over more extended periods (for example, recalling movements associated with a particular song from week to week).

P3 (ii) pupils use emerging conventional communication.

* They greet known people and may initiate interactions and activities (for example, performing an action such as clapping hands to initiate a particular song).
* They can remember learned responses over increasing periods of time and may anticipate known events (for example, a loud sound at a particular point in a piece of music).
* They may respond to options and choices with actions or gestures (for example, choosing a shaker in a rhythm band activity).
* They actively explore objects and events for more extended periods (for example, tapping, stroking, rubbing or shaking an instrument to produce various effects).
* They apply potential solutions systematically to problems (for example, indicating by eye contact or gesture the pupil whose turn it is to play in a 'call and response' activity).

P4 pupils use single words, gestures, signs, objects, pictures or symbols to communicate about familiar musical activities or name familiar instruments.

* With some support, they listen and attend to familiar musical activities and follow and join in familiar routines.
* They are aware of cause and effect in familiar events (for example, what happens when particular instruments are shaken, banged, scraped or blown, or that a sound can be started and stopped or linked to movement through a sound beam).
* They begin to look for an instrument or noisemaker played out of sight.
* They repeat, copy and imitate actions, sounds or words in songs and musical performances.

P5 pupils take part in simple musical performances.

* They respond to signs given by a musical conductor (for example, to start or stop playing).
* They pick out a specific musical instrument when asked (for example, a drum or a triangle).
* They play loudly, quietly, quickly and slowly in imitation.
* They play an instrument when prompted by a cue card.

They listen to, and imitate, distinctive sounds played on a particular instrument.

They listen to a familiar instrument played behind a screen and match the sound to the correct instrument on a table.

P6 pupils respond to other pupils in music sessions.

They join in and take turns in songs and play instruments with others.

They begin to play, sing and move expressively in response to the music or the meaning of words in a song.

They explore the range of effects that can be made by an instrument or sound maker.

They copy simple rhythms and musical patterns or phrases.

They can play groups of sounds indicated by a simple picture or symbol-based score.

They begin to categorise percussion instruments by how they can be played (for example, striking or shaking).

P7 pupils listen to music and can describe music in simple terms (for example, describing musical experiences using phrases or statements combining a small number of words, signs, symbols or gestures).

They respond to prompts to play faster, slower, louder, softer.

They follow simple graphic scores with symbols or pictures and play simple patterns or sequences of music.

Pupils listen and contribute to sound stories, are involved in simple improvisation and make basic choices about the sound and instruments used.

They make simple compositions (for example, by choosing symbols or picture cue cards, ordering them from left to right, or making patterns of sounds using computer software).

P8 pupils listen carefully to music.

They understand and respond to words, symbols and signs that relate to tempo, dynamics and pitch (for example, faster, slower, louder, higher and lower).

They create their own simple compositions, carefully selecting sounds.

They create simple graphic scores using pictures or symbols.

They use a growing musical vocabulary of words, signs or symbols to describe what they play and hear (for example, fast, slow, high, low).

They make and communicate choices when performing, playing, composing, listening and appraising (for example, prompting members of the group to play alone, in partnership, in groups or altogether).

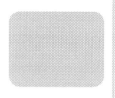

Bibliography

Anderson, A. (2020a) *The Schumann frequency and 5G.* Available online at https://www.linkedin.com/pulse/schumann-frequency-5g-ange-anderson/?trackingId=Iqal3WxE3dnKLlM4OpjY9g%3D%3D.

Anderson, A. (2020b) *Therapeutic Trampolining for Children and Young People with Special Educational Needs: A practical Guide to Supporting Emotional and Physical Wellbeing.* Routledge.

Sensory Education (n.d.) Research on Auditory Integration Training (AIT). Available online at auditoryintegrationtraining.co.uk/auditory-integration-training-ait-for-hearing-autism-adhd-add-dyslexia-and-other-special-needs-2/clinical-studies-for-auditory-integration-training/.

Beauchene, C., Abaid N., Moran R., Diana, R.A. and Leonessa, A. (2017) The Effect of Binaural Beats on Verbal Working Memory and Cortical Connectivity. *J Neural Eng.* April, 14(2): 026014.

Beecham, T. (1978) *Beecham Stories: Anecdotes, Sayings and Impressions of Sir Thomas Beecham,* 1st edn. Robson Books.

Bryan, J. (2018) *Eye Can Write.* Lagom Publishers.

Cirelli, L., Jurewicz, Z. and Trehub, S. (2019) Effects of maternal singing style on mother–infant arousal and behavior. https://doi.org/10.1162/jocn_a_01402.

Clayton, M., Sager, R. and Will, U. (2004) *In Time with the Music: The Concept of Entrainment and Its Significance for Ethnomusicology.* ESEM CounterPoint, Vol. 1.

Cody, J. (1996) *Infrasound.* Available online at https://borderlandsciences.org/journal/vol/52/n02/Cody_on_Infrasound.html.

Dolman, G. (2005) *What to Do About Your Brain-Injured Child.* Square One Publishers.

Einstein, A. (n.d.) https://quotefancy.com/quote/762846/Albert-Einstein-Future-medicine-will-be-the-medicine-of-frequencies, and https://www.goodreads.com/quotes/7603-if-i-were-not-a-physicist-i-would-probably-be.

Emoto, M. (2006) *Water Crystal Healing: Music and Images to Restore Your Wellbeing.* Beyond Words Publishing.

Engagement Model (2020) Available online at https://www.gov.uk/government/publications/the-engagement-model.

Estyn (2015) Available online at https://www.estyn.gov.wales/thematic-reports/best-practice-teaching-and-learning-creative-arts-key-stage-2-may-2015.

Fitch, W.T. (2009) *Musical Protolanguage: Darwin's Theory of Language Evolution Revisited.* Available online at https://www.languagelog.ldc.upenn.edu.

Goodwin, T.J. (2003) *Physiological and Molecular Genetic Effects of Time-Varying Electromagnetic Fields on Human Neuronal Cells.* Available online at https://ntrs.nasa.gov/archive/nasa/casi.ntrs.nasa.gov/20030075722.pdf.

Greene, B. (2000) *The Elegant Universe: Superstrings, Hidden Dimensions and the Quest for the Ultimate Theory*. Vintage.

Griffiths, G.M., Hastings, R.P., Williams, J. et al. (2019) Mixed Experiences of a Mindfuless-Informed Intervention: Voices from People with Intellectual Disabilities, Their Supporters and Therapists. *Mindfulness*, 10: 1828–1841. https://doi.org/10.1007/s12671-019-01148-0.

Grisham, J. (2016) *The Tumour*, 3rd edn. Focused Ultrasound Foundation.

Halberg, O. and Oberfield, G. (2006) Will We All Become Electrosensitive? *Electromagnetic Biology and Medicine*, 25: 189–191. Available online at Criimen.org.

Hellmuth Margulis, E. (2018) *The Psychology of Music: A Very Short Introduction*. Oxford University Press.

Jacobi, E., Richter, O. and Krüskemper, G. (1981) Simulated VLF-Fields as a Risk Factor of Thrombosis. *International Journal of Biometeorology*, 25(2): 133–142.

Jirakittayakorn, N. and Wongsawat, Y. (2017) *Brain Responses to a 6-Hz Binaural Beat: Effects on General Theta Rhythm and Frontal Midline Theta Activity*. Available online at https://pubmed.ncbi.nlm.nih.gov/28701912/.

Jonas, S. (2011) Available online at https://www.innerharmonyhealthcenter.com/parkinsons-research.

Juliano, A.C., Alexander, A.O., DeLuca, J. and Genova, H. (2020) Feasibility of a School-Based Mindfulness Program for Improving Inhibitory Skills in Children with Autism Spectrum Disorder. *Research in Developmental Disabilities*, 101: 103641. DOI: 10.1016/j.ridd.2020.103641.

Kepler, J., with Aiton, E.J., Duncan, A.M. and Field, J.V. (trans.) (1997) *The Harmony of the World*. American Philosophical Society.

Lakhovsky (1925) Available online at https://multiwaveoscillator.com/articles/mwocuringcncr.htm.

Le Scouarnec, R.P., Poirier, R.M., Owens, J.E., Gauthier, J., Taylor, A.G. and Foresman, P.A. (2001) Use of Binaural Beat Tapes for Treatment of Anxiety: A Pilot Study of Tape Preference and Outcomes: *Altern Ther Health Med*. January, 7(1): 58–63.

Leventhall, G. (2009) Low Frequency Noise. What We Know, What We Do Not Know, and What We Would Like to Know. *Journal of Low Frequency Noise, Vibration and Active Control*, 28(2). Available online at https://waubrafoundation.org.au/wp-content/uploads/2013/04/Leventhall-LFN-Whatweknow.pdf.

Levitin, D. (2019) *This is Your Brain on Music: Undrstanding a Human Obsession*. Penguin Books.

Lundqvist, L., Andersson, G. and Viding, J. (2009). Effects of Vibroacoustic Music on Challenging Behaviors in Individuals with Autism and Developmental Disabilities. *Research in Autism Spectrum Disorders*, 3(2): 390–400. DOI: 10.1016/j.rasd.2008.08.005.

Lutz, F. and Andeweg, H. (1995) *Resonance Therapy in Eight Steps*. Institute for Resonance Therapy, Cappenberg, Germany.

Lynes, B. (1987) *The Cancer Cure that Worked*. Marcus Books.

Munroe Institute (n.d.) Available online at https://www.monroeinstitute.org/blogs/free-meditations.

Ockelford, A. (2009) Zygonic Theory: Introduction, Scope, and Prospects. *ZGMTH* 6(1): 91–172. https://doi.org/10.31751/400.

Ockelford, A., Welch, G. and Zimmermann, S. (2002) Focus of Practice: Music Education for Pupils with Severe or Profound and Multiple Difficulties – Current Provision and Future Need. *British Journal of Special Education*, 29(4): 178–182.

Oster, G. (1973) Auditory Beats in the Brain. *Scientific American*, 229(4): 1073–1094. Available online at www.amadeux.net/sublimen/documenti/G.OsterAuditoryBeatsintheBrain.pdf.

Porges, S.W., Bazhenova, O.V., Bal, E., Carlson, N., Sorokin, Y., Heilman, K.J., Cook, E.H. and Lewis, G.F. (2014) Reducing Auditory Hypersensitivities in Autistic Spectrum Disorder: Preliminary Findings Evaluating the Listening Project Protocol. *Front Pediatr.*, August, 1(2): 80. DOI: 10.3389/fped.2014.00080.

PROMISE (2015) Available online at https://www.researchgate.net/publication/306959911_The_Provision_of_Music_in_Special_Education.

RfL (2019) Available online at https://hwb.gov.wales/curriculum-for-wales/routes-for-learning/.

Rossignol, D.A. and Frye, R. (2011) Melatonin in Autism Spectrum Disorders: A Systematic Review and Meta-Analysis. *Journal of Developmental Medicine & Child Neurology*, 53(9): 783–792.

Saroka, K.S., Caswell, J.S., Lapointe, A. and Persinger, M.A. (2014) Greater Electroencephalographic Coherence between Left and Right Temporal Lobe Structures During Increased Geomagnetic Activity. *Neuroscience Letters*, 560: 126–130.

Skille, O. (2007) Available online at vibroacoustic.org/FrequencyInfo/Research%20Articles/Reports. Olav%20Skille.pdf.

Skille, O. (2013) Available online at https://www.olavat.com.

Somatron (n.d.) Available online at http://www.somatron.com/music.html.

Soundbeam (n.d.) Available online at http://www.soundbeam.co.uk/vibroacoustic/downloads/what-is-vibroacoustic-therapy.pdf

Stacy, R., Brittain, K. and Kerr, S. (2002) Singing for Health: An Exploration of the Issues. *Health Education*, 102(4): 156–162.

Stehli, A. (1995) *The Sound of a Miracle*. Beaufort Books.

Successful Futures (2015) Available online at gov.wales.publications.

Tesla, N. (2014) *High Frequency Oscillators for Electro-Therapeutic and Other Purposes* (ebook). Sublime Books.

Tolle, E. (2009) *A New Earth*. Penguin.

Vickhoff, B., Malmgren, H., Åström, R., Nyberg, G., Ekström, S.R., Engwal, M., Snygg, J., Nilsson, M. and Jörnsten, R. (2013) Music Structure Determines Heart Rate Variability of Singers. *Frontiers in Psychology Journal*. Available online at https://doi.org/10.3389/fpsyg.2013.00334.

Vladimirsky, B.M., Sidyakin, V.G., Temuryanz, N.A., Makeev, V.B. and Samokhvalov, V.P. (1995) Cosmos and biological rhythms. Eupatoria City Typography, Simferopol: 77–111.

Wigram, A. (1995) *Current List of Contraindications for Vibroacoustic Therapy*. Radlett: Horizon NHS Trust. Unpublished.

Winder, K.C. (2020) Joining a Choir Helped Me Combat Anxiety and Find a Meditative State of Pure Joy. *The Guardian*. Available online at theguardian.com/lifestyle/2020/jan/13.

Zentner, M. and Eerola, T. (2010) *Rhythmic Engagement with Music in Infancy*. PNAS. Available online at https://doi.org/10.1073/pnas.1000121107.

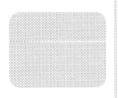

Index

Printed in the United States
by Baker & Taylor Publisher Services